AF572755

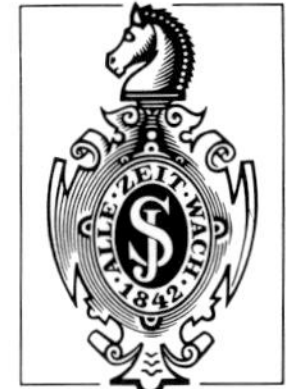
ALLE ZEIT WACH
1842

# Critical Leg Ischaemia
## Its Pathophysiology and Management

Edited by
John A. Dormandy and Günter Stock

With 27 Figures

Springer-Verlag Berlin Heidelberg New York
London Paris Tokyo Hong Kong

John A. Dormandy

Department of Vascular Surgery
St. George's Hospital
and Medical School
London, England

Günter Stock

Research Laboratories
Schering AG, Berlin
Federal Republic of Germany

ISBN 3-540-52462-2 Springer-Verlag Berlin Heidelberg New York
ISBN 0-387-52462-2 Springer-Verlag New York Heidelberg Berlin

Library of Congress Cataloging-in-Publication Data
Critical leg ischaemia: its pathophysiology and management/edited by John A. Dormandy and Günter Stock.
p. cm.
ISBN 0-387-52462-2 (U.S. alk. paper)
1. Peripheral vascular diseases. 2. Leg – Blood-vessels – Diseases. 3. Ischemia. I. Dormandy, J. A. II. Stock, G. (Günter) [DNLM: 1. Ischemia – management. 2. Ischemia – physiopathology. 3. Leg – blood supply. WE 850 C934] RC694.C75 1990 617.5′8 – dc20 DNLM/DLC



Typesetting, printing and bookbinding: Brühlsche Universitätsdruckerei, Giessen
2125/3020-543210 – Printed on acid-free paper

# Preface

*Jean Natali*

The pathophysiology and management of chronic critical limb ischaemia (CLI) has always been a problematic area, at least partly because it involves doctors from a wide range of the traditional medical specialities including vascular surgery, angiology, diabetology, haematology and radiology. The treatment of these patients also varies largely with local circumstances and national traditions. CLI therefore seemed a particularly appropriate subject for a new type of European consensus approach.

In 1988 a series of small workshops were held by the European Working Group on Critical Limb Ischaemia to discuss the definition, pathophysiology, investigation and management of this condition. The process culminated in a meeting in Berlin in March, 1989 where 120 specialists from sixteen European countries, representing the basic sciences as well as a spectrum of clinical disciplines, met to evolve a Consensus Document on the subject with specific recommendations. The Document, which is reproduced in the first section of this book, does not of course necessarily represent the unanimous view of all those who participated in its compilation; however it is agreed that it does represent a consensus or majority view. It was also noted that the comments and recommendations in the document should be taken as a whole, and are not intended to dictate the only correct approach to individual treatment. The Document has been widely discussed, reviewed and served as a basis for a plenary session on Critical Limb Ischaemia at the International Union of Angiology meeting in September 1989. Acute limb ischaemia was not considered in this consensus process.

However the Document is only an amalgamation or summary of a large number of expert opinions and does not include detailed arguments or a review of the existing literature. It was therefore thought useful to expand it into a book with individual chapters, written by experts in the various specialities concerned in the consensus process. In general, chapters are followed by a commentary, written by a specialist in a different discipline, looking at the same topic from a different point of view. This approach illustrates the multidisciplinary aspect of the management of these patients and it is hoped that, not only will it stimulate further examination of the whole subject, but provide practising doctors everywhere with a new insight into this difficult and demanding condition. (Cross references to specific recommendations in the Consensus Document are indicated in the margin of the text in the individual chapters.) The Consensus process itself will continue and, after individual European societies have met and examined the recommendations from their own perspective, representatives from all the societies will meet together in 1991 to distil a new and refined Consensus Document II.

*"Any fool can cut off a leg; it takes a surgeon to save one",*
George C. Ross (1834–1892)

*"Any fool can cut off a leg, but it takes a social worker, nurse counsellor, non-invasive flow technician, radiologist, laser expert, surgeon, hospital administrator and medical defence lawyer to save one".*
Adrian Marston
(English surgeon)

# European Consensus Document on Critical Limb Ischaemia

March 1989

# 1. Definition and epidemiology of chronic critical limb ischaemia

*Recommendation 1:* It is recommended that all units dealing with critical limb ischaemia should maintain accurate audited records of patients treated and their progress.

## 1.1 Basic definition

Critical limb ischaemia is ischaemia which endangers the limb or part of a limb. Acute ischaemia should be distinguished from chronic ischaemia, and will not be discussed in this document.

*Recommendation 2A:* Critical limb ischaemia is defined by the following two criteria:

persistently recurring rest pain requiring regular analgesia for >2 weeks

and/or ulceration or gangrene of the foot or toes

plus ankle systolic pressure <50 mmHg*

* Calcification of the arteries in diabetes and other diseases makes measurement of the ankle pressure unreliable – absent palpable pulses are sufficient for definition of critical limb ischaemia in diabetics and patients with calcified arteries.

*Recommendation 2B:* A more precise definition is required for published reports or for the design and reporting of clinical trials. In addition to the above definition, further evidence of ischaemia has to be obtained by angiography and/or one of the following tests:

- toe systolic blood pressure <30 mmHg
- transcutaneous oxygen pressure of the ischaemic area ($tcPO_2$) $\leqslant$10 mmHg and which does not increase with inhalation of oxygen
- absence of arterial pulsations in big toe (measured with strain gauge or photoplethysmography after vasodilatation)
- marked structural or functional changes of the skin capillaries in the affected area.

The relevance of these additional measurements should be quantified by prospective studies looking at the specificity and sensitivity of each test in terms of predicting prognosis.

*Fontaine classification*

In practice, the Fontaine classification can be slightly altered to correspond with the above definition of critical limb ischaemia. All patients with Fontaine stage IV disease (ulceration or gangrene) have critical limb ischaemia as well as those patients with stage III disease (rest pain) and ankle pressure less than 50 mmHg. Therefore if stage III is subdivided into:

- stage $III_A$ rest pain + ankle pressure above 50 mmHg
- stage $III_B$ rest pain + ankle pressure below 50 mmHg

both patients with stage IV and stage $III_B$ disease can be said to have critical limb ischaemia (*NOT STAGE* $III_A$).

## 1.2 Incidence and prevalence

There is little information available on the incidence and prevalence of critical limb ischaemia. However, it is estimated that the prevalence of peripheral arterial disease in the whole population is 5% in men aged over 50 and less than 10% of these will ever develop critical limb ischaemia.

Diabetes predisposes to the development of critical limb ischaemia, and diabetics are over 5 times more likely to develop critical limb ischaemia than non-diabetics. In secondary and tertiary referral centres specialising in circulatory problems in diabetics, approximately 20% of diabetic patients have critical limb ischaemia; however, this figure is inflated by referral of the most difficult cases.

In Denmark, for example, there are 300 amputations per year in 100000 diabetics compared with 1400 amputations per year in the total non-diabetic population (5000000). However, some of the amputations in diabetics may be performed for lesions of neuropathic rather than ischaemic origin, thereby overestimating the incidence of critical limb ischaemia. The prevalence of diabetes varies from about 2% of the population in Denmark to about 5% of the population in Spain. Type I diabetes is more common in northern than in southern Europe. The incidence of type I diabetes varies from 29.5/100000/year in Finland to 4.4/100000/year in France.

The only statistical data available which indicate the prevalence of critical limb ischaemia are the number of amputations performed. On the assumption that all amputations are performed for ischaemia and only 25% of patients with critical limb ischaemia ever have an amputation, multiplication of this figure by four gives an approximation of the number of patients with critical limb ischaemia. The numbers of referrals to limb-fitting centres also give an estimate of the number of amputations, although probably no more than half of all amputees are referred for limb fitting.

Using the above assumption and the amputation rates in Table 1, the incidence of critical limb ischaemia is approximately 500–1000/million population/year.

**Table 1.** Incidence of major amputation in the population

| Estimated incidence | Source |
|---|---|
| 120/million/yr | Experience of district hospitals in the UK |
| 200/million/yr | Referrals to limb-fitting centres in the UK |
| 260/million/yr | Veterans Administration, USA |
| 300/million/yr | Amputation rate extrapolated from the Framingham study |
| 320/million/yr | Danish hospital survey |

## 1.3 Current prognosis/fate

There is little hard data concerning the fate of patients with critical limb ischaemia. In diabetic patients with critical limb ischaemia, the immediate treatment is amputation in about 20%, about a further 20% undergo percutaneous transluminal angioplasty (PTA), about 15% undergo surgical reconstruction, and there is no genuinely appropriate immediate treatment for the remaining 45%. The immediate fate of a mixed group of patients presenting with chronic critical limb ischaemia would be approximately 60% undergoing a vascular reconstruction, 20% primary amputation and 20% some other form of temporary treatment. A year later 25% will have had a major amputation, 55% will still have two legs and 20% will be dead.

Patients with rest pain and ulceration have a worse prognosis than patients with rest pain and no ulceration. There is no difference in the prognosis of patients with small or more extensive ulcers; patients with any size of ulcer or with gangrene have a poor prognosis irrespective of ankle pressure. Patients with only rest pain who have an ankle pressure of less than 40 mmHg have a worse prognosis than those with an ankle pressure greater than 40 mmHg.

Patients with critical limb ischaemia have a poor survival. In the United States approximately 50% of amputees survive for 3 years. Cardiovascular disease is the usual cause of death in these patients.

# 2. Pathophysiology of critical limb ischaemia

The pathophysiology of critical limb ischaemia in humans remains to be established. The following view is merely a hypothesis considered most likely by the participants, but much of it is based on the extrapolation of results from animal studies.

## 2.1 Macrocirculation

Atherosclerosis of the large arteries is the fundamental process in the pathogenesis of critical limb ischaemia. Atherosclerosis occluding or severely narrowing the proximal conducting arteries reduces blood flow and perfusion pressure to the more distal circulation, giving a reduced flow to the microcirculation. This is the primary problem in critical limb ischaemia and leads to the microcirculatory changes described below.

Platelets and leucocytes may become activated as they pass over an ulcerated atherosclerotic plaque and post-stenotic vortices in the proximal arteries, thereby perfusing the limb with activated platelets and leucocytes.

## 2.2 Microcirculation

The microcirculation comprises the arterioles, venules and capillaries. Skin microvessels can be subdivided into thermoregulatory and nutritional capillaries; the latter carrying only 15% of total flow.

It is controversial whether all arterioles in the critically/ischaemic area are already maximally dilated. There may be normal morphological capillary density, but there is a reduced functional capillary density. This is combined with capillary dilatation, low red cell velocity and microthrombi. Some capillaries show normal perfusion, but low flow velocity. There is significantly delayed appearance of Na-fluorescein and reduced $tcPO_2$.

### *2.2.1 Techniques for evaluating skin microcirculation*

New techniques which have recently improved understanding of the skin microcirculation include:

- $tcPO_2$ measurement
- laser-Doppler flux measurement
- capillaroscopy – fluorescence
  – morphological
  – dynamic
- combinations of the above.

### *2.2.2 Vasomotion*

Vasomotion – the rhythmic distribution of flow to the capillaries – is abnormal in patients with critical limb ischaemia with or without diabetes. There may be reduction in low frequency flow motion waves (3–12/min) and an increase in high frequency flow motion waves (approx. 20/min). Abnormal vasomotion produces maldistribution of blood flow with some capillaries not perfused or underperfused.

Studies show that in patients with Fontaine stage III and IV PAOD, there is abnormal vasomotion which can be quantified by frequency and amplitude analysis. So called small wave (high frequency and low amplitude) flux motion occurs in patients with PAOD, but only occasionally in healthy patients. These waves are abolished after successful PTA.

### *2.2.3 Vasospasm*

The role of vasospasm in the pathogenesis of critical limb ischaemia is controversial, although there is evidence in animals that blood flow patterns may be altered by constriction of the precapillary arterioles. Although there is no direct clinical evidence, vasospasm may be mediated by endothelium-derived constricting factors (EDCF), and favoured by lack of endothelium-derived relaxing factor (EDRF) and prostacyclin ($PGI_2$). Platelet and leucocyte-derived substances, e.g. thromboxane $A_2$ ($TXA_2$), leukotrienes and serotonin (5HT), may also promote vasoconstriction.

### *2.2.4 Haemorheology*

Rheological factors alone may promote maldistribution of blood flow and exacerbate the detrimental effects of other factors, e.g. blockage by platelet aggregates.

Besides blood pressure, the main determinants of blood flow in the normal circulation are haematocrit, blood cell deformability and plasma viscosity. Leucocytes and erythrocytes have diameters of about 7–8 μm and nutritive capillaries have diameters of about 3–15 μm. Therefore, leucocytes and erythrocytes must deform to pass through the nutritive capillaries. In the normal circulation under high shear stress and high perfusion pressures, leucocytes and erythrocytes deform easily, although leucocytes are much more rigid. In critical limb ischaemia, there is a pronounced fall in the perfusion pressure and blood flow rate. Due to the drop in perfusion pressure, erythrocytes and particularly leucocytes deform less readily and passage through nutritive capillaries is more difficult.

There is increased erythrocyte aggregation and release of adenosine diphosphate in critical limb ischaemia. Bulk viscosity of blood increases and erythrocyte deformability is decreased due to acidosis, hyperosmolarity and calcium accumulation. Fibrinogen levels are elevated in critical limb ischaemia which further increases plasma viscosity and erythrocyte aggregation, leading to poor perfusion. Fibrinogen levels are increased by smoking, diabetes and infection.

Leucocytes and platelets are activated by the altered shear stresses. Trapping of leucocytes and platelet aggregates occurs and further impairs blood flow in the microcirculation. This further favours leucocyte-vessel wall interactions, worsens blood flow and exacerbates ischaemia.

Many of these rheological changes, such as increased viscosity, haematocrit and plasma fibrinogen are predictors of poor prognosis in patients with critical limb ischaemia.

## 2.3 Microvascular flow regulating system (MFRS) and microvascular defence system (MDS) and their breakdown in critical limb ischaemia

All the factors which have been discussed in the preceding sections on physiology and pathophysiology can be considered in terms of an overall concept of MFRS and MDS.

### *The normal circulation*

#### Microvascular flow regulating system (MFRS)

The MFRS regulates and distributes blood flow in the normal microcirculation (see Figure 1). It is characterised by normal vasomotion, with regular, periodic perfusion of capillary networks. Microcirculatory flow is influenced by EDRF and one or more endothelium-derived constricting factors.

#### Microvascular defence system (MDS)

In health, the MDS consists of an appropriate interaction of the platelets, leucocytes and endothelium as a defensive reaction to injury and infection (see Figure 2).

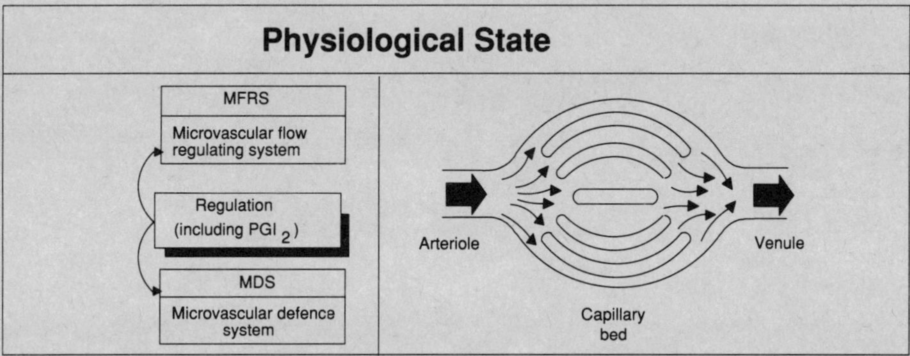


**Fig. 1.** Diagrammatic representation of normal microcirculatory physiology

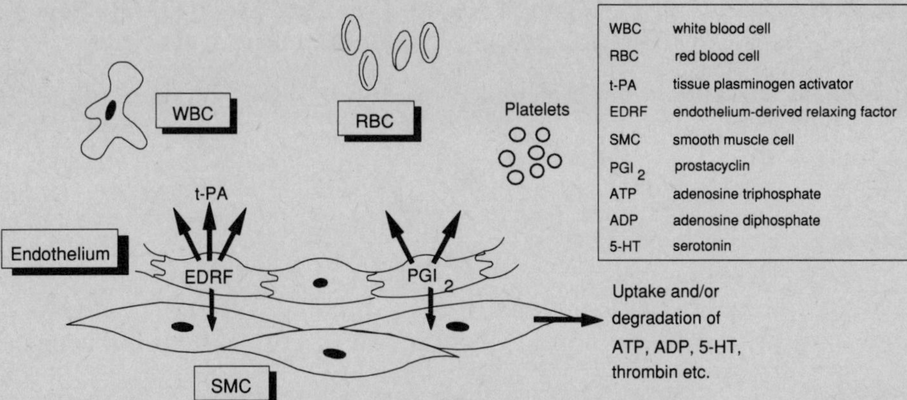


**Fig. 2.** Components of Microvascular Defence System (MDS) under normal physiological conditions. The blood cells (WBC, RBC, platelets) are under physiological conditions in a non-adhering, non-secretory state.

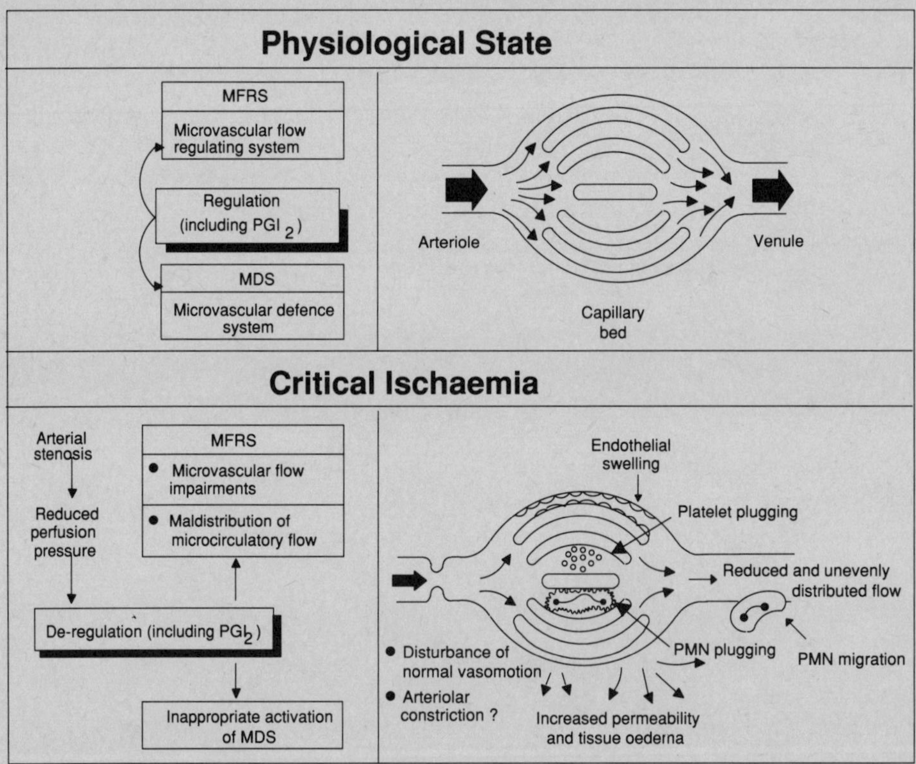


**Fig. 3.** Hypothesis of overall microcirculatory changes associated with critical limb ischaemia. PMN, polymorphonuclear leucocyte; MDS, microvascular defence system; MFRS, microvascular flow regulating system

*Critical limb ischaemia*

Breakdown of MFRS

In critical limb ischaemia there is breakdown of the MFRS, principally due to the decrease in the arterial perfusion pressure, with maldistribution of blood flow in the microcirculation, especially the nutritive skin capillaries (see Figure 3). Theoretically, there may be constriction of precapillary arterioles and the balance between EDRF and EDCF shifting in favour of the latter. In addition, activated platelets and leucocytes release vasoconstrictor substances, e.g. leukotrienes, $TXA_2$ and 5-HT.

Breakdown of MDS

In critical limb ischaemia there is inappropriate activation of the MDS, with activation of leucocytes and platelets, and damage to the endothelium. This is always associated with local hypoxia and metabolic changes, and may be triggered by trauma, systemic metabolic changes such as diabetes and infection. Inappropriate activation of the MDS results in vicious cycles between the activated leucocyte, the activated platelet and the damaged endothelium. The difference between endothelial cell injury and activation is still unclear (see Figures 4 and 5).

In addition, there is release of growth factors by the endothelium, macrophages and platelets which stimulate proliferation of vascular smooth muscle. Endothelial swelling, platelet plugging, leucocyte plugging and tissue oedema occur in this inflammatory reaction.

Prostacyclin ($PGI_2$)

In the normal microcirculation, $PGI_2$ plays an important role in the regulation of the MFRS and the MDS. $PGI_2$ has antithrombotic, leucocyte- and endothelium-stabilising properties, can modulate the previously mentioned vicious cycles and can maintain patency of capillaries and dilate small and larger vessels. $PGI_2$ is currently viewed as being of prime importance in normalising the MFRS and deactivating the MDS in critical limb ischaemia.

## 2.4 Special features of diabetes

The pathophysiology of critical limb ischaemia in diabetics differs from that in non-diabetics in that the abnormalities already described are further exaggerated in diabetic patients. The presence of autonomic neuropathy in diabetics not only alters the clinical signs and symptoms of the disease, but also complicates the pathophysiology. In addition, there are further functional disturbances in the diabetic microcirculation.

*Macroangiopathy vs. microangiopathy*

Diabetic vascular disease can be divided morphologically into three groups: disease of the large arteries (macroangiopathy), disease of the small arteries and

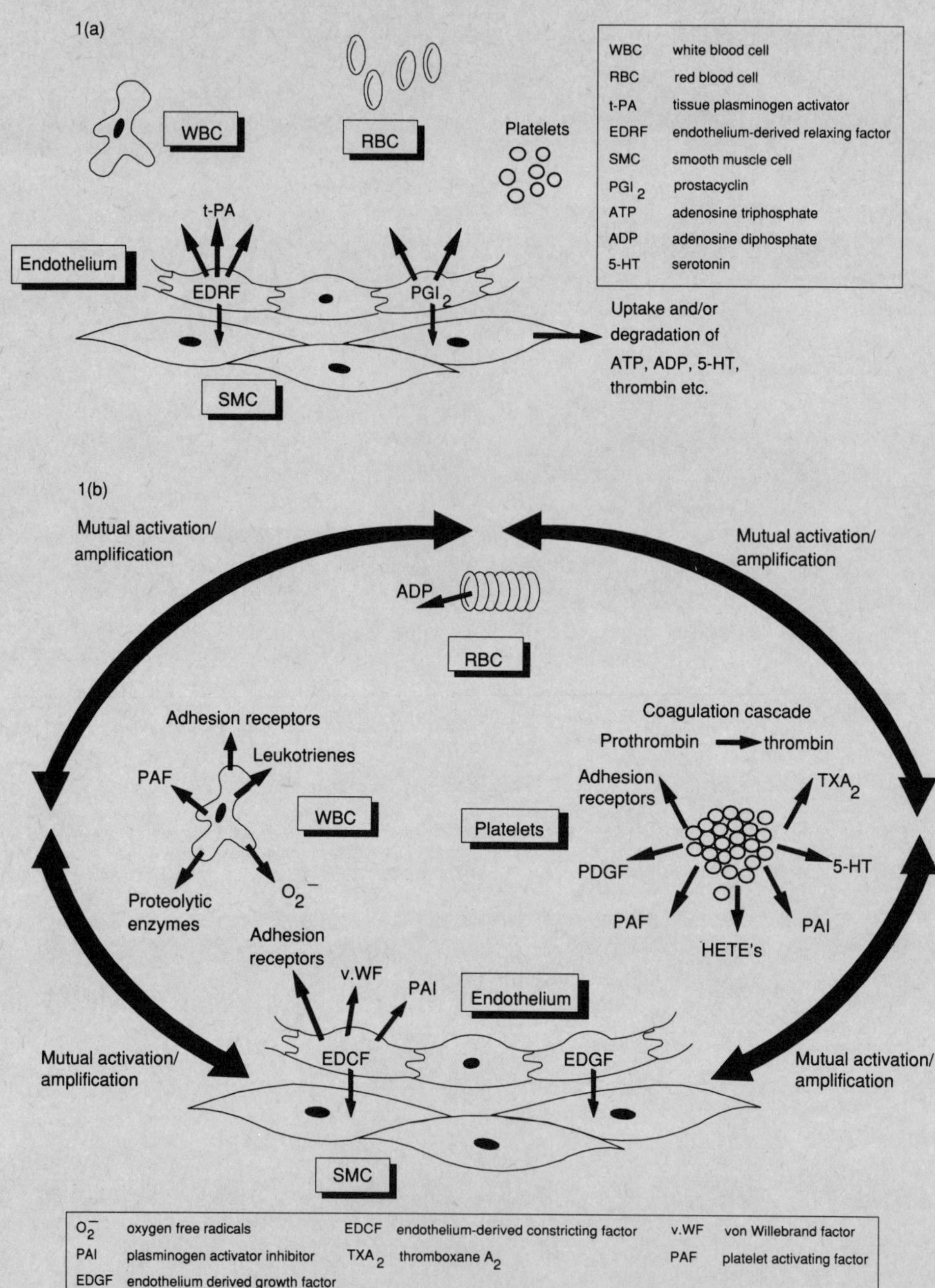


**Fig. 4.** Components of Microvascular Defence System (MDS) under physiological conditions (1 a) and under pathophysiological conditions as is likely to occur in critical limb ischaemia (1 b). The blood cells (WBC, RBC, platelets) are under physiological conditions in a non-adhering, non-secretory state.

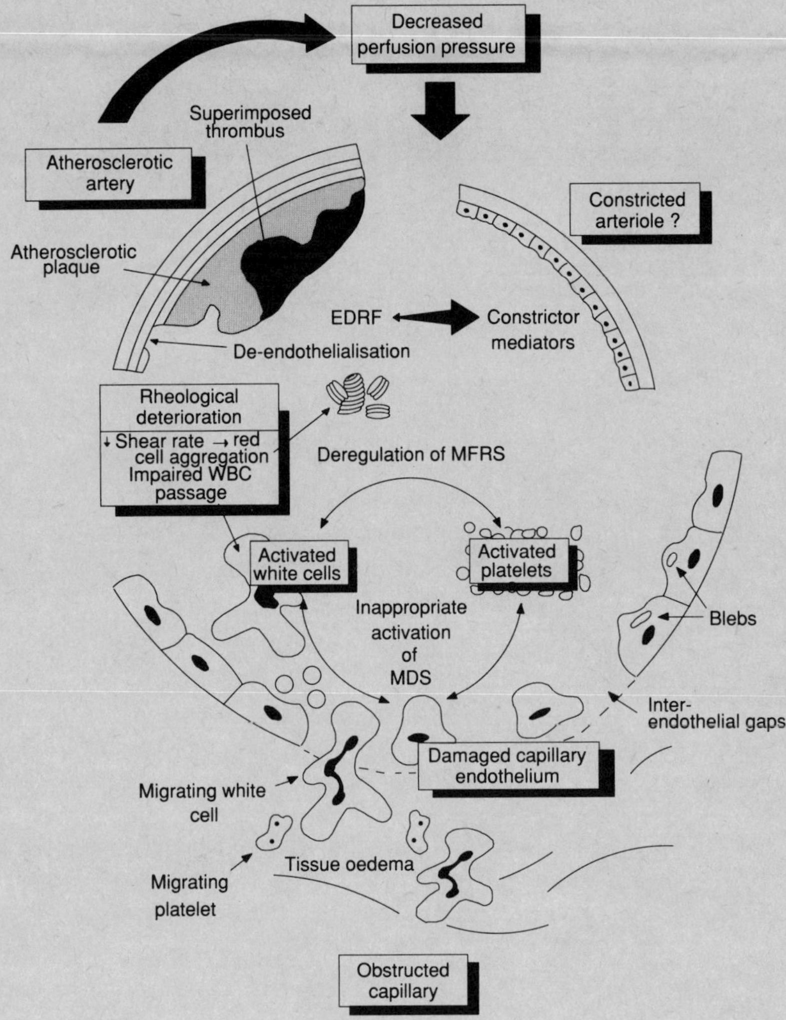


**Fig. 5.** Summary of suggested pathophysiological changes in critical limb ischaemia at different levels of the circulation

arterioles and capillary disease (microangiopathy). The site of large vessel disease in diabetics is usually more distal than in non-diabetics. In addition, the disease site appears to differ between type I and type II diabetic patients. There is controversy as to whether the pathology of atherosclerosis differs in diabetics and non-diabetics.

### *Loss of veno-arteriolar reflex*

In diabetics there may be a loss of the veno-arteriolar reflex on standing, causing tissue oedema which may further impair the microcirculation.

*Vasomotion*

In the poorly-controlled diabetic patient there are abnormalities of vasomotion even in the absence of critical limb ischaemia. These abnormalities may be normalised by good control of blood glucose levels.

*Blood components*

The following abnormalities are exaggerated in diabetic compared with non-diabetic patients with critical limb ischaemia:

- increased platelet adhesion and aggregation
- increased adhesion of blood components to the endothelium
- reduced $PGI_2$ production by the endothelium
- greater release of oxygen free radicals by leucocytes
- lowered fibrinolytic activity
- thickening of the capillary basement membrane and impaired passage of leucocytes
- reduced EDRF release
- reduced erythrocyte deformability
- functional microcirculatory abnormalities
- increased capillary permeability.

*Immunological changes*

The immune system is altered in diabetic patients; antibodies may be glycosylated and their function altered. Poorly controlled diabetics are more prone to infection than well-controlled diabetics. Bacterial growth is inhibited by lactic acid, but in the presence of diabetic ketosis this inhibition of bacterial growth is blocked.

Overall, the presence of ketosis and hyperglycaemia in poorly-controlled diabetics increases the vicious cycles in the pathogenesis of critical limb ischaemia.

# 3. Assessment, investigation and general management of patients with critical limb ischaemia

## 3.1 Assessment and investigations

### *3.1.1 Minimum necessary investigations*

A full clinical history and examination should be performed.

In diabetes, examination should include full neurological testing (including pain, temperature and touch sensation, vibration sense and reflexes).

> ***Recommendation 3:*** The following investigations are recommended in all patients presenting with critical limb ischaemia:
>
> Cardiovascular system
> - resting ECG
> - chest X-ray
>
> Macrocirculation
> - segmental blood pressure measurement (unreliable in diabetics due to media sclerosis of the arteries – oscillography should be used)
> - angiography (abdominal aorta to foot) or digital subtraction angiography (DSA) using arterial injection.
>
> Blood tests
> - full blood count
> - ESR or plasma viscosity
> - serum creatinine
> - blood sugar
> - electrolytes
> - platelet count
> - liver enzymes
> - prothrombin time
> - fibrinogen
>
> Bacteriology if appropriate
> - culture and sensitivities

### *3.1.2 Additional optional investigations*

***Recommendation 4:*** The following further investigations are recommended in all patients with critical limb ischaemia, if the facilities to perform these tests are available and appropriate:

*Cardiovascular system*
- exercise ECG (if facilities exist for exercise not involving the legs)

*Macrocirculation*
- Doppler waveform analysis of the peripheral arteries
- Doppler scan of carotids
- duplex scanning

*Microcirculation*
- $tcPO_2$ measurement at varying levels in the leg
- capillaroscopy
- laser-Doppler fluxmetry

*Blood tests*
- cholesterol
- triglycerides
- HDL
- protein electrophoresis
- 24-hour blood sugar profile
- $HbA_1$ or $HbA_1c$

The following investigations may be useful in diabetic patients:
- toe systolic blood pressure
- pulse volume
- X-ray of the foot
- bone scan

## 3.2 General management

A high proportion of patients with critical limb ischaemia have other co-existent diseases, especially cardiovascular and renal disorders. Lung disease, such as chronic bronchitis or bronchial carcinoma, often occurs due to the high proportion of smokers in the patient population. **Patients must be told to stop smoking.** There may be co-existent local and systemic infection. These concomitant diseases may render the patients unsuitable for surgery, general anaesthesia or even angiography.

### *3.2.1 Other overt co-existent cardiovascular disease*

Coronary heart disease

Up to 90% of patients with critical limb ischaemia have been shown to have coronary heart disease on coronary angiography.

***Recommendation 5:*** Before arterial surgery, the possibility of the patient requiring coronary bypass surgery should be borne in mind. Patients with severe cardiac symptoms and/or a positive exercise ECG should be referred for specialist opinion.

Hypertension

An elevated blood pressure in the early phase of critical limb ischaemia helps to improve perfusion of the affected limb. However, hypertension increases the incidence of cardiovascular complications. Therefore a difficult balance has to be maintained to ensure adequate perfusion of the limb and limit the risk of stroke. Beta-blockers may have a deleterious effect on peripheral blood flow.

***Recommendation 6:*** Antihypertensive treatment should not be instituted in the early stage of critical limb ischaemia in patients whose systolic blood pressure in the standing or sitting position is lower than 180 mmHg and diastolic blood pressure lower than 100 mmHg.

If the patient is on antihypertensive drugs and has a blood pressure well below the above mentioned levels, the possibility of reducing or discontinuing treatment during the initial management of critical limb ischaemia should be considered. An increase of the systemic blood pressure by 10–20 mmHg may produce a similar pressure increase in the ischaemic area with a possible improvement of the ischaemic symptoms.

If treatment of hypertension is necessary, angiotensin converting enzyme (ACE) inhibitors, calcium antagonists or other vasodilating substances should be used. Do not use beta-blockers.

Heart failure and arrhythmia

***Recommendation 7:*** Heart failure and arrhythmias should be treated, taking care not to reduce the blood pressure too far.

### *3.2.2 Infection*

Antibiotics may be required systemically in patients who have ulcers or gangrene and clinical evidence of spreading infection. Systemic antibiotics may be administered intravenously, but in some countries are administered intra-arterially as this is believed to produce higher tissue concentrations. The risk of gas gangrene and infection spreading quickly in the critically ischaemic limb should be borne in mind.

***Recommendation 8:*** Systemic antibiotic administration is recommended in patients with clinical evidence of infection, but should not be used routinely in all patients to avoid inducing bacterial resistance. Systemically administered antimycotic agents may be required, in addition to antibiotics, if there is proven evidence of fungal infection.

### *3.2.3 General management of the ischaemic limb*

Patients with critical limb ischaemia involving necrosis require rest with protection of the affected part of the limb. Downward tilting of the foot of the bed may be beneficial and the affected limb should be in the lowest possible position without inducing oedema. Any ulceration or necrosis should be kept dry with mechanical removal of necrotic tissue and drainage of pus.

***Recommendation 9:*** Patients with necrosis should have the limb placed in the lowest possible position without oedema formation.

### *3.2.4 Diabetes*

(Only the general management of the diabetic patients is discussed in this section, the specific treatment of the diabetic foot is discussed in section 5.2.)

***Recommendation 10:*** Patients with purely neuropathic disease should be clearly differentiated from those with neuroischaemic disease because the management of the patient will be different. A large proportion of pure neuropathic ulcers can be healed with rest or the use of casting and appropriate treatment of the infection.

Table 2 is a guide to the differentiation between pure neuropathic and neuroischaemic lesions. In practice this can sometimes be very difficult.

**Table 2.** Differentiation of neuropathic and neuroischaemic ulcers

| Neuropathic ulcer | Neuroischaemic ulcer |
|---|---|
| palpable pulses<br>increase in total blood flow<br>loss of small fibre sensation* before loss of large fibre sensation**<br>presence of plethysmographically-detectable pulsations | absence of pulses<br>decrease in total blood flow<br>loss of large fibre sensation** before loss of small fibre sensation*<br>absence of plethysmographically-detectable pulsations |

* small fibre sensation is pain/temperature
** large fibre sensation is touch/vibration

Management of the diabetic patient

*1. Management of the acute problem.*
Prompt treatment of dehydration and infection is particularly important in diabetics.

*Treatment of oedema and control of blood sugar.* In diabetic patients especially, capillary permeability is increased leading to oedema. Treatment with diuretics may be advantageous to remove the oedema and so improve the microcirculation by reducing interstitial pressure. In such cases, treatment for several months may be required.

***Recommendation 11:*** Blood sugar should be normalised as far as possible (at least <200 mg/dl) and practically all patients with critical limb ischaemia should be converted to insulin. Patients should be rehydrated, if required. Where necessary, oedema should be treated with a non-thiazide diuretic, taking care to maintain normal potassium levels.

*Role of angiography.* Where conservative treatment is possible in diabetic patients, angiography may be delayed for 2 to 4 weeks. During this time neuropathic ulcers in diabetic patients may heal with conservative treatment. There is an increased incidence of renal failure in diabetic patients and angiography should be performed with caution.

***Recommendation 12:*** Angiography should be performed in diabetic patients, even with clinically neuropathic lesions, if there is no improvement after 2 weeks of medical treatment.

*Purely neuropathic ulcers.* Conservative treatment of neuropathic ulcers produces good results in over 90% of cases.

*Treatment of infection.* The indications for selective antibiotic use are when there is clinical evidence of infection of the foot. Antibiotics are administered after obtaining a swab from the ulcer and discontinued once there are no clinical signs of infection.

*2. Preventive treatment.*
*Prevention of recurrence of ulceration in diabetic patients.*

Education of the diabetic patient is important to prevent the recurrence of ulcers and gangrene. Prophylactic measures include the provision of suitable footwear, chiropody, regular visits to the diabetic clinic, as well as educating patients to examine their feet regularly.

*Preventive treatment by management of risk factors*

***Recommendation 13:*** To try to prevent the recurrence of complications in diabetic patients the following targets for good control are recommended:

**Table 3.** Targets for optimal control in both type I and type II diabetics

| | |
|---|---|
| Blood glucose | |
| fasting | 80–120 mg/dl |
| postprandial | 80–160 mg/dl |
| $HbA_1$ | Normal |
| Urine glucose | None |
| Total cholesterol | <200 mg/dl |
| HDL-cholesterol | >40 mg/dl |
| Fasting triglycerides | <150 mg/dl |

The target levels in the above table are intended primarily for younger patients.

It is even more important to treat the risk factors (including hyperinsulinism) in diabetic patients than in non-diabetics. Smoking is an even more adverse risk factor in diabetic patients than in non-diabetics; diabetics should therefore be especially encouraged to give up smoking. Regular exercise is also to be encouraged in diabetics.

### *3.2.5 Team approach*

Whether a patient is referred by the general practitioner to a general physician, angiologist, diabetologist or surgeon may be influenced by local factors: which specialist group mainly deals with critical limb ischaemia in that country, the type of patient and the general practitioner's expectation of treatment (i.e. whether there appears to be the option of surgery, medical treatment or PTA).

Ideally, there should be a combined approach to the treatment of patients between surgeons, angiologists, other internists and interventional radiologists. Co-operation between angiologists or radiologists and surgeons is required when performing PTA, since the presence of a surgeon on stand-by is required in case of complications with the procedure. In practice, there is often co-operation between angiologists, other physicians and surgeons in discussing problem patients who are controversial.

A slightly different team of specialists may be involved in the diabetic patient: the diabetologist (or physician), vascular surgeon, dermatologist, nurse, chiropodist, plaster technician, shoe fitter, physiotherapist, limb fitter and social worker.

***Recommendation 14:*** Close co-operation between disciplines is particularly desirable in the management of both diabetic and non-diabetic patients with critical limb ischaemia.

# 4. Specific treatment of the ischaemic limb

## 4.1 Percutaneous catheter procedures

These procedures carry a lower mortality and morbidity than surgical techniques, and may therefore be applicable even in patients unfit for surgery or as an adjunct to surgery. They are performed by different specialists depending upon local practice and expertise: for example, angiologists, interventional radiologists and surgeons.

### *4.1.1 Angioplasty*

Techniques and indications

The available techniques comprise PTA, laser-assisted PTA, the use of various new catheters and perioperative angioplasty. A combination of PTA and thrombolysis can be performed in special cases. PTA is ideal in single or multiple short stenoses, but is also suitable for treatment of occlusions up to approximately 10 cm. PTA can be used in combination with reconstructive surgery, for instance, in a combination of femoropopliteal graft with perioperative dilatation of a short iliac stenosis. It is also sometimes performed as a final alternative to amputation in patients totally unfit or unsuitable for reconstructive surgery.

Disadvantages

1. About 3% of patients who undergo PTA will require urgent surgery due to complications.
2. There is a risk of embolization with PTA, particularly near the aortic bifurcation. However, most of the emboli can be treated by local thrombolysis at the same session.

Contraindications

The contraindications to PTA are:

- thrombosed peripheral aneurysms
- bleeding disorders.

However, these contraindications apply to few patients considered for PTA.

The main limiting factors are:

- sharply kinked arteries
- calcified arteries
- obesity.

Results

PTA is successful in up to 95% of iliac stenoses and up to 90% of femoral stenoses or short occlusions, with a 3-year patency rate of 85% and 60%, respectively.

*Recommendation 15:* PTA is recommended in patients with stenoses or short occlusions, following discussion with vascular surgeons and angiologists. PTA may also be considered as an attempt at limb salvage in patients unsuitable for vascular reconstruction and likely to require an amputation.

### *4.1.2 Local thrombolysis by direct infiltration with or without percutaneous transluminal angioplasty (PTA)*

*Technique.* Local thrombolysis delivers directly to the arterial occlusion lower doses of urokinase or streptokinase than systemic thrombolysis. It is widely believed that lysable material may be present for up to 12 months after thrombus formation in the iliac artery, for up to 6 months in the superficial femoral artery and for up to 1 month in the crural region.

Contraindications and limiting factors are similar to those pertaining to PTA.

*Advantages.* The dose of thrombolytic agent is considerably reduced when it is applied locally. Hence, the side effects are much less with local thrombolysis than with systemic thrombolysis. Whereas systemic thrombolysis is contraindicated after recent surgery, local thrombolysis is possible within 2 or 3 days of surgery.

*Recommendation 16:* Local thrombolysis with or without PTA is recommended in:

- acute-on-chronic occlusions of proximal arteries within the time limits given above
- distal infrapopliteal occlusions within the time limits given above
- bypass grafts occluded by thrombus.

The duration of symptoms is a reliable guide to the age of the thrombus.

*Recommendation 17* (General recommendation for all forms of catheter procedures): All trainee vascular surgeons, interventional radiologists and angiologists should spend some time familiarising themselves with these techniques in an experienced unit.

*Recommendation 18:* PTA should only be performed in centres where vascular surgical facilities are available.

### *4.1.3 Pharmacological prophylaxis after successful cathether procedures*

*Rationale for therapy.* Catheter procedures cause damage to the vascular wall. During the acute event there is release of potentially harmful factors, and a thrombogenic surface is formed.

PTA alone

*Current therapy.* On a theoretical basis, a number of drugs could be used following PTA to prevent reocclusion, including the oral anticoagulants, antiplatelet drugs, dextran, some Ca antagonists and prostanoids. Of these, so far only salicylate has been shown to be effective and this only after PTA in the coronary arteries.

In practice, salicylate is usually given before the intervention and continued for 3 to 12 months post-intervention.

> ***Recommendation 19:*** On theoretical and clinical grounds, salicylate is recommended after PTA of stenoses and short occlusions. Treatment should be continued for at least one year, and longer in the absence of side effects if there are any residual lesions.

Local thrombolysis alone or in combination with PTA.

> ***Recommendation 20:*** Heparin and overlapping oral anticoagulant therapy is recommended following local thrombolysis alone or in combination with PTA. The same regimen should be followed after PTA of long occlusions. Treatment should be continued for at least one year, or longer in the presence of any residual lesions.

## 4.2 Surgical procedures

### *4.2.1 Limb salvage reconstructions*

Reconstructive surgery is indicated in patients with critical limb ischaemia, where there is evidence of sufficient run-off.

Short grafts show better patency than long grafts, and graft patency is reduced with prosthetic grafts compared with autologous vein grafts. There is no good evidence at present showing a difference in patency between reversed and in situ autologous vein grafts.

Disadvantages

Early failure of reconstructive surgery may worsen the ischaemia and result in amputation at a higher level than would otherwise be necessary. If the procedure fails, there is an increased mortality from the combined surgical procedure and amputation.

Follow-up

Approximate patency rates of reconstructive procedures at different levels are shown in the following table:

**Table 4.** Approximate 1-year patency rates for reconstructive procedures

| Operation | 1-year patency |
|---|---|
| Aorto-ilio-femoral | 95% |
| Femoro-popliteal AK (vein) | 85% |
| Femoro-popliteal AK (prosthetic) | 80% |
| Femoro-popliteal BK (vein) | 80% |
| Femoro-popliteal BK (prosthetic) | 70% |
| Femoro-proximal tibial (vein) | 70% |
| Femoro-distal tibial (vein) | 55% |
| Femoro-proximal tibial (prosthetic) | 50% |
| Femoro-distal tibial (prosthetic) | 25% |

AK = above knee, BK = below knee

Graft occlusion is usually caused by thrombosis. Graft failure may be related to the flow properties of blood through the vessel. Greater graft length increases the occlusion rate, increased diameter decreases the flow velocity and hence increases the occlusion rate. There is a higher incidence of graft failure with prosthetic materials than with autologous vein grafts.

Graft patency is not necessarily equivalent to limb salvage. With time, there is a greater discrepancy between graft patency and limb salvage due to collateral formation and late graft failure may not affect the viability of the leg. Amputation is required more frequently for early than for late graft failures, thus the longer a graft stays open, the lower the chances of amputation.

***Recommendation 21:*** A reconstructive procedure should be attempted so long as there is a reasonable chance of saving a useful limb in a patient who has evidence of sufficient run-off and is fit for surgery.

### *4.2.2 Management of graft failure*

Reasons for early graft failure:

Essentially early graft failure may be due to:
1. Incorrect choice of operation (e.g. ignoring a proximal or distal obstruction)
2. Technical error at the time of operation (which can be largely avoided by perioperative angiograms)
3. Combination of other factors which cannot be specified or influenced.

Reasons for late graft failure

Late graft failure is due to progression of the disease or hyperplasia of the pseudo-intima at the anastomoses.

Prevention of graft failure

Evaluation of grafts before they fail and prevention of failure is better than attempting to salvage the limb after graft failure. Frequent evaluation of grafts during the first year may help to prevent failure and improve the 5-year patency rate by up to 20%. Ideally new strictures should be treated before they progress to complete occlusion.

> ***Recommendation 22:*** Infra-inguinal grafts should be regularly evaluated during the first year to anticipate failure.

Therapeutic options following graft failure

When a first reconstruction has failed, the following therapeutic options are available:

- a further attempt at reconstructive surgery
- thrombolysis of the occluded graft
- surgical thrombectomy
- indirect procedures – sympathectomy<br>profundoplasty
- medical therapy
- amputation.

> ***Recommendation 23:*** Graft patency should be confirmed at the end of surgery. Following early graft failure, re-exploration should only be undertaken when there is a reasonable chance of restoring patency.

> ***Recommendation 24:*** Following late graft failure patients with critical limb ischaemia should be considered for interventional catheter procedures or further surgery.

### *4.2.3 Amputation*

Level of major amputations

Because of the lower morbidity and mortality, below knee (BK) amputation is preferred to above knee (AK) if at all possible.

Amputees have a very poor prognosis, both in terms of rehabilitation and survival. Only 70% of BK amputations heal primarily, another 15% heal by second intention and 15% require AK amputation. A major amputation on the other leg is required in 30% of cases. The hospital mortality of BK and AK amputations is 8% and 18%, respectively. Approximately 40% of amputees will be dead within two years of their first major amputation. Full mobility is only ever achieved in

50% of BK and 25% of AK amputations. Whilst the ratio of BK to AK amputations is increasing in some countries, in many others it has not changed for the last 20 years.

The case for primary amputation

In some cases, primary amputation may be better than subjecting the patient to repeated surgical procedures with little chance of success and increasing mortality and morbidity. This can be a very difficult decision where a team approach may be particularly useful.

> ***Recommendation 25:*** Primary amputation should only be undertaken if the possibility of revascularisation procedures has been excluded.

> ***Recommendation 26:*** Amputations should be followed by appropriate rehabilitation.

### *4.2.4 Sympathectomy*

Surgical sympathectomy or chemical sympathectomy, with phenol or absolute alcohol, may be performed in patients with critical limb ischaemia. The number of surgical sympathectomy procedures performed has decreased in the last two decades.

Sympathectomy is currently sometimes used in the following circumstances:

- thrombotic occlusions of digital arteries
- as a last resort in intractable rest pain where there is no possibility of a surgical reconstruction
- thromboangiitis obliterans (TAO).

Advantages/disadvantages

Surgical sympathectomy may be longer lasting than chemical sympathectomy, but must be performed under general anaesthesia. In some patients with critical limb ischaemia, sympathectomy may lead to warming of the foot and some subjective improvement, but there is no good evidence that it alters the ultimate fate of the patient. Chemical sympathectomy in particular may improve the symptoms of critical limb ischaemia.

Although combining a reconstructive operation with lumbar sympathectomy may be logical, in that the latter may improve run-off, controlled trials have failed to confirm any benefit from the additional sympathectomy.

> ***Recommendation 27:*** Sympathectomy alone has never been shown to improve limb salvage in critical limb ischaemia, but may be the treatment of last resort for alleviation of rest pain.

### 4.2.5 *Nerve stimulation*

Spinal cord stimulation may relieve pain, and additionally may increase skin blood flow, but there are insufficient data to make a recommendation.

### 4.2.6 *Post-surgical pharmacotherapy*

Reconstructive surgery

There is a considerable variation in current treatment after reconstructive surgery: either no pharmacological treatment, antiplatelet drugs, anticoagulants or dextran-40, depending upon individual practice and national variations. There are few conclusive trials showing that any of these therapies prevent recurrence, although there is a theoretical justification for most.

***Reccommendation 28:*** No pharmacological therapy is required following reconstructive surgery above the inguinal ligament.

***Recommendation 29:*** Following reconstructions below the inguinal ligament, some form of drug therapy may be useful to reduce graft failure, but its effectiveness still remains to be proven.

## 4.3 Primary pharmacotherapy

***Recommendation 30:*** There is little evidence available for the efficacy of oral anticoagulants, other forms of anticoagulation, antiplatelet drugs, vasoactive drugs or fibrinogen-lowering drugs in the treatment of chronic critical limb ischaemia. It is possible, but not formally proven, that oral and non-oral anticoagulant drugs may prevent macro- or micro-thromboembolic events in these patients. Similarly these drugs may also prevent the progression of peripheral arterial occlusive disease.

$PGI_2$, $PGI_2$-analogues and $PGE_1$

Considering the prostacyclins act favourably on activated platelets, activated leucocytes and leucocyte-vessel wall interactions, damaged endothelium and microvascular perfusion and integrity, it would seem that they act on almost all components believed to be responsible for failure of the microvascular flow-regulating system, secondary to the reduction in perfusion pressure. By this multifactorial effect on the interactive vicious circle sustaining microvascular ischaemia, prostacyclins may reinstitute the MFRS and thereby provide the prerequisites for ischaemic tissue healing. Other modes of action may be involved.

There is some evidence that intra-arterial $PGE_1$ may be effective in patients with critical limb ischaemia. Several chemically stable derivatives of $PGI_2$ have been synthesised and are currently being investigated for the treatment of critical limb ischaemia. There are controlled clinical trials in patients with critical limb ischaemia unsuitable for reconstructive surgery or other catheter procedures, in which ulcer healing appears to improve.

***Recommendation 31:*** Some clinical trials support the recommendation that treatment with $PGI_2$, $PGI_2$-analogues and $PGE_1$ should be considered in patients with critical limb ischaemia unsuitable for reconstructive surgery or PTA, except in those who require immediate amputation.

## 4.4 Isovolaemic haemodilution

The haematocrit is frequently elevated in patients who are heavy smokers. There is no controlled clinical trial showing the benefit of isovolaemic haemodilution alone in critical limb ischaemia, although there is a theoretical basis for isovolaemic haemodilution as an adjunct to reconstructive surgery. There is no agreement on the level of haematocrit at which isovolaemic haemodilution should be performed or the target haematocrit to which it should be reduced. In addition, dehydrated patients should be rehydrated.

***Recommendation 32:*** The benefit of isovolaemic haemodilution is not proven, however, if the haematocrit remains $>50$ despite cessation of smoking and rehydration, haemodilution may be considered.

# 5. Choice of primary treatment and general treatment plan

## 5.1 Thromboangiitis obliterans (TAO)

It is difficult to differentiate TAO from atherosclerotic peripheral vascular disease, but the following criteria are normally used:

1) mostly male, aged under 50, heavy smokers
2) normal proximal arteries with distal occlusions only
3) "corkscrew" collaterals distally
4) absence of classical risk factors for atherosclerosis
5) frequent thrombophlebitis migrans
6) frequent upper limb involvement.

The incidence of TAO is greater in Mediterranean and Asian countries than in Northern Europe.

Reconstructive surgery is usually impossible in patients with TAO. Sympathectomy is frequently performed in TAO and is said to be useful in early disease. There is virtually no experience with PTA in TAO, since the technique is not available in many of the countries where the disease is most prevalent. In the acute stage of the disease, immunosuppressive therapy has been shown to be useful.

> ***Recommendation 33:*** Patients with TAO must stop smoking and undertake physical activity in the chronic stage when the wounds are healed. A trial of pharmacological therapy should be undertaken as reconstructive surgery is rarely helpful. A sympathectomy can be useful.

## 5.2 The diabetic foot

The following recommendations are specific to the care of the critically-ischaemic foot in diabetic patients. They are in addition to those considered for non-diabetics.

The purely neuropathic foot

About 90% of purely neuropathic ulcers heal with routine medical treatment, hence these patients should be differentiated from those with neuroischaemic disease. Even in apparently totally neuropathic ulcers, which do not heal after about two weeks of medical treatment, angiography should be performed to evaluate the need and feasability of PTA or surgery.

The neuroischaemic foot

Surgery and PTA are possible in a smaller proportion of diabetics than non-diabetics with critical limb ischaemia because the disease is more distal. In diabetics, there are problems in ascertaining whether there is a patent vessel in the foot on angiography. Some surgeons explore the foot and look for a suitable vessel, whilst others perform an amputation if no patent vessels are visible on angiography.

***Recommendation 34:*** Diabetic patients with neuropathic ulcers and foot pulses may need non-invasive assessment and/or angiography. Early drainage of pus or debridement may be required as reconstructive surgery and PTA are rarely appropriate or possible. Local treatment and appropriate footwear will usually suffice.

***Recommendation 35:*** Diabetic patients with ulcers or gangrene and absent foot pulses should have an angiogram performed before amputation is considered.

## 5.3 Aortic disease

### *5.3.1 Stenoses*

Although aortic stenoses alone rarely cause critical limb ischaemia, either PTA or surgery may be used. The role of PTA in the aorta is controversial.

***Recommendation 36:*** Surgery is the treatment of choice in stenosis of the abdominal aorta causing critical limb ischaemia particularly if embolization is suspected.

### *5.3.2 Occlusions (long/short)*

Although aortic occlusions rarely cause critical limb ischaemia, good results are usually obtained with reconstructive surgery for aortic occlusions, but this is a relatively major procedure.

***Recommendation 37:*** Surgery is the procedure of choice for aortic occlusions, provided the patient is reasonably fit for major surgery. If unfit, extra-anatomic procedures might be acceptable.

***Recommendation 38:*** Where there is multilevel disease and haemodynamically significant arterial occlusion, treatment of the proximal lesion alone is usually sufficient.

## 5.4 Iliac disease

### *5.4.1 Stenoses*

These are ideal cases for PTA. Series from specialised centres report reopening rates in iliac stenoses of up to 95% and a 3-year patency rate of up to 85%. PTA should be avoided in patients with long, irregular, bilateral iliac stenoses or in curved arteries, where surgery may be more appropriate.

> ***Recommendation 39:*** PTA is the procedure of choice in most cases of iliac stenosis.

### *5.4.2 Occlusions*

Reconstructive surgery is applicable in most cases, although for short occlusions (up to 5 cm), PTA can be used effectively. Local thrombolysis in the iliac arteries can be dangerous. In the future laser-assisted PTA may play a greater role in occluded vessels than PTA alone.

> ***Recommendation 40:*** Reconstructive surgery is the treatment of choice in most cases of iliac occlusive disease, although PTA can be used for short (less than 5 cm) occlusions.

## 5.5 Femoro-popliteal disease

### *5.5.1 Stenoses*

An isolated stenosis of the femoral artery rarely causes critical limb ischaemia.

> ***Recommendation 41:*** Single or multiple short stenoses of the superficial femoral and popliteal arteries, especially with multilevel disease, can cause critical limb ischaemia and should be treated initially by PTA alone.

### *5.5.2 Occlusions*

If the origin of the profunda is occluded, local reconstruction of the profunda femoris may be sufficient. In superficial femoral occlusion sufficiently severe to warrant surgery, either an in situ or reversed vein femoro-popliteal bypass may be appropriate.

Angioplasty with or without thrombolysis may be performed, or laser-PTA used for lesions up to 30 cm. A combination of intraoperative angioplasty and an in situ graft is a further alternative in this location.

*Recommendation 42:* In critical limb ischaemia, a vein bypass is recommended for long AK occlusions.

## 5.6 Predominantly distal (below knee) disease

Below the knee, vein grafts should also be used where possible. If necessary, a composite graft with PTFE may be used as an alternative to amputation. Alternatives to long prosthetic grafts to the ankle should be found where possible.

Tibial procedures are worthwhile, and although long-term patency may be poor, procedures above the ankle may offer a chance to avoid amputation. Despite variable results, procedures to the peroneal artery may provide equally good results as those to the anterior and posterior tibials.

The lower limit of PTA is controversial, different centres producing different results.

*Recommendation 43:* In distal disease with resonable run-off, surgery using autologous vein is probably the procedure of choice.

*Recommendation 44:* Prosthetic grafts to the ankle vessels or below rarely succeed, however, they might still be indicated as an alternative to amputation.

*Recommendation 45:* Before amputation is thought of in patients with distal disease, PTA or pharmacotherapy should be considered.

## 5.7 Place of primary medical treatment

There is little or no good evidence that existing oral vasoactive drugs are beneficial in critical limb ischaemia, but there have been some good results with parenteral prostanoids. Ineffective drugs are not placebos – they may have adverse effects.

In all patients, the following recommendation applies:

*Recommendation 46:* Primary medical treatment for critical limb ischaemia can be used when reconstructive surgery or catheter procedures:

- are not technically possible
- are contraindicated
- carry an unacceptable risk/benefit ratio

however, more clinical trials of pharmacotherapy need to be performed.

# Conclusions

There is much progress still to be made in our understanding and treatment of critical limb ischaemia. In particular:

1. The multidisciplinary approach and expertise available in relatively few centres should be made more widely available. This applies particularly to the rapid advances which have been made in various percutaneous catheter procedures.

2. Despite these advances, and the recent tendency for more distal bypass grafts, a proportion of patients with critical limb ischaemia still require a major amputation either as a primary procedure, but more often after a series of failed attempts at limb salvage.

3. There is clearly a need for an effective pharmacological treatment for the many patients unsuitable or unfit for either a percutaneous catheter or reconstructive procedure, or in patients where these procedures have failed.

4. The same rigorous standards should be applied to trials of percutaneous catheter procedures or surgical techniques as are generally applied to drug therapy. Large controlled trials are required for the proper evaluation of all therapies.

# Meeting Attendees

Adar R
Department of Vascular Surgery
Sheba Medical Center
Tel-Hashomer 52621
Israel

Allenberg JR
Chirurg. Univ.-Klinik Heidelberg
Sektion Gefäßchirurgie
Im Neuenheimer Feld 110
D-6900 Heidelberg 1
FRG

Andreani D
Institute of 2nd Medical Clinic
University of Rome "la Sapienza"
Policlinico Umberto 1
Roma
Italy

Andreassian B
Hôpital Beaujon
100 Boulevard du Général Leclerc
92118 Clichy Cedex
France

Balas P
4 Hiraclitou Street
Athens 10673
Greece

Barros D'Sa AAB
Vascular Surgery Unit
Royal Victoria Hospital
Grosvenor Road
Belfast BT126BA
UK

Bartolo M
Via Nazionale 230
00184 Roma
Italy

Becquemin JP
Hôpital Henri Mondor
51 avenue de lattre de tassigny
9400 Créteil
France

* Bell P
Department of Surgery
Clinical Sciences Building
Leicester Royal Infirmary
Leicester LE2 7LX
UK

Bergqvist D
Department of Surgery
Malmö General Hospital
S-21401 Malmö
Sweden

Biasi GM
Divisione di Chirurgia Vascolare
Ospedale E Bassini
Via Massimo Gorki 50
20092 Cinisello Balsamo
Milano
Italy

Boccalon H
Hôpital Rangueil
31054 Toulouse Cedex
France

Boisseau MR
Hémobiològie
Hôpital Cardiologique
33604 Pessac
France

* Bollinger A
Department of Internal Medicine
Medical Policlinic Angiology
Division
University Hospital
CH-8091 Zürich
Switzerland

Bouchier-Hayes D
Department of Surgery
Beaumont Hospital
Beaumont Road
Dublin 9
Eire

Boulton AJM
Department of Medicine
Manchester Royal Infirmary
Oxford Road
Manchester M13 9WL
UK

Branchereau A
Service de Chirurgie Vasculaire
Hôspital La Timone
13385 Marseille Cedex 4
France

Braquet P
Institut Henri Beaufour
17 Avenue Descartes
F-92350 Le Plessis Robinson
France

Breddin K
Center of Internal Medicine
Division of Angiology
JW Goethe-University
Theodor-Stern-Kai 7
D-6000 Frankfurt am Main 70
FRG

Catalano M
Clinica Medica Generale e Terapia Medica
Universitá degli Studi di Milano
c/o Ospedale L Sacco
via GB Grassi 74
20157 Milano
Italy

Cathelineau G
Hôpital Saint-Louis
1 Rue Claude Vellefaux
75010 Paris
France

Chant AB
Amberley
Braishfield
Romsey
Hants SO51 0PR
UK

Chiariello M
Clinica Medica I
c/o Nuovo Policlinico
II Universita'
Via Pansini 5
80131 Napoli
Italy

Clement D
Akademisches Ziekenhuis
Dienst Inw Ziekten
De Pintelaan 185
B-9000 Gent
Belgium

Clyne AC
Level 5, Vascular Unit
Torbay Hospital
Lawes Bridge
Torquay
Devon TQ2 7AA
UK

Coget J
61 Rue de Turenne
59000 Lille
France

Connor H
The County Hospital
Hereford HR1 4ER
UK

Courbier R
Fondation Hôpital Saint-Joseph
26 Boulevard de Louvain 13285
Marseille Cedex 8
France

Creutzig A
Zentrum f Inn Med/Abt Angiologie
Med Hochschule
Podbielskistraße 380
3000 Hannover 51
FRG

D'Addato M
Cattedra di Chirurgia Vascolare
Policlinico S Orsola
Via Massarenti 9
40138 Bologna
Italy

Davi G
Via Marchese UGO 52
90141 Palermo
Italy

De Gaetano G
Centro di Ricerche Biomediche
E Farmacologiche
66030 Santa Maria Imbaro
Italy

De Sobregrau RC
c/Capellades 342a
08023 Barcelona
Spain

Diehm C
Medizinische Universitätsklinik
Bergheimer Straße 58
D-6900 Heidelberg
FRG

* Dormandy JA
St James Wing
St Georges' Hospital
London SW17 0QT
UK

Dzsinich C
Clinic of Cardiovascular Surgery
Városmajor u68
1122 Budapest
Hungary

Edmonds ME
Diabetic Department
Kings College Hospital
Denmark Hill
London SE5 9RS
UK

Ehringer H
1 Med Universitätsklinik
Angiologische Abteilung
Lazarettgasse 14
A-1090 Vienna
Austria

Eikelboom B
Department of Surgery
St Antonius Hospital
3435 CM Nieuwegein
The Netherlands

* Fagrell B
Department of Medicine
Karolinska Hospital
S-10401 Stockholm
Sweden

Federlin K
Medizinische Klinik III und
Poliklinik der Justus-Liebig-
Universität
Rodthohl 6
D-6300 Giessen
FRG

Fernandes e Fernandes J
Department of Vascular Surgery
Hospital Santa Maria
Av Prof Egas Moniz
Lisboa
Portugal

Fiessinger JN
Service de Médecine Interne et de
Pathologie Vasculaire
Hôpital Broussais
96 Rue Didot
75674 Paris Cedex 14
France

Forbes C
Department of Medicine
Ninewells Hospital
Dundee DD1 9SY
UK

Franco A
Centre Hospitalier Universitaire
38043 Grenoble Cedex
France

Franzeck UK
Dept of Internal Medicine
Universitätshospital
Rämistraße 100
CH-8091 Zürich
Switzerland

Garcia-Robles R
Hospital Ramón y Cajal
Servicio de Endocrinología
Carretera de Colmenar KM 9.100
28034 Madrid
Spain

Gruss JD
Kurhessisches Diakonissenhaus
Abt Gefäßchirurgie
Goethestr 85
3500 Kassel
FRG

Guilmot JL
CHU Bretonneau
Clinique Medicale B
37044 Tours
France

Hagen B
Chefarzt der Radiologie
Martin Luther Krankenhaus
Caspar Theyss Straße 27
1000 Berlin 33
FRG

Harris P
The Vascular Surgery Unit
Ward 25
Broadgreen Hospital
Thomas Drive
Liverpool L14 3LB
UK

Held K
Chefarzt der Inneren Abteilung
Ev Krankenhaus Göttingen-Weende
An der Lutter 24
3400 Göttingen
FRG

Hild R
Medizinische Klinik
Franz Josef Krankenhaus
Landhausstraße 25
D-6900 Heidelberg
FRG

Horrocks M
Bristol Royal Infirmary
Marlborough Street
Bristol BS2 8HW
UK

Housley E
Clinic for Peripheral Vascular
Diseases
Royal Infirmary
Edinburgh EH3 9YW
Scotland

Janbon C
Clinique Medicale B
Hôpital Saint-Eloi
Avenue Bertinsans
34000 Montpellier
France

Janka HU
Schwabing City Hospital
III Med Abt
Kölner Platz 1
D-8000 München 40
FRG

Jantet G
41 Audley Road
London W5 3ES
UK

Jeans WD
Department of Radiodiagnosis
Bristol Royal Infirmary
Marlborough Street
Bristol BS2 8HW
UK

Kniemeyer H
Abt f Gefäßchirurgie und
Nierentransplantation
Chirurgische Universitätsklinik
Moorenstr 5
D-4000 Düsseldorf
FRG

Kitslaar P
Academisch Ziekenhuis
Sint Annadal 1
6214 PA Maastricht
The Netherlands

Kretschmer G
1st Surgical Clinic
University of Vienna
Alserstraße 4
A-1090 Vienna
Austria

* Krone W
Room 500
5th Floor Medical Clinic
University Hospital Eppendorf
Hamburg
FRG

Larroque P
Hôpital Begin
Service de Pathologie Cardiovasculaire
69 Avenue de Paris
94160 Saint Mande
France

Le Devehat C
Unité de Recherches
d'Hémorhéologie
Clinique – Centre de Diabetologie
Centre Hôpitalier de Nevers
58320 Pougues les Eaux
France

Libretti A
Clinica Medica Generale
Università degli Studi di Milano
c/o Ospedale L Sacco
Via GB Grassi 74
20157 Milano
Italy

Lowe G
Glasgow Royal Infirmary
Department of Medicine
10 Alexandra Parade
Glasgow G31 2ER
UK

Lucchesi B
The University of Michigan
Medical School
Medical Science Building I-M6322
Department of Pharmacology
Ann Arbor
48109 Michigan
USA

Mahler F
Angiologische Abteilung
Universitäts Hospital
CH-3010 Berne
Switzerland

Mashiah A
Vascular Surgery Unit
Kaplan Hospital
Rehovot 76100
Israel

Matesanz JM
Dept Angiologia y Cirugia Vascular
Hospital Clinical san Carlos
C/Dr Martin Lagos, s/n
Universidad Complutense
28015 Madrid
Spain

Maurer PC
Head of Dept of Vascular Surgery
Technical University of Munich
Medical School
Rechts der Isar Medical Center
Ismanigerstraße 22
8000 Munich 80
FRG

Mehta J
Box J-277
JHMHC
Department of Medicine
Gainesville
Florida 32610
USA

Mercier C
Hôspital de la Conception
Rue Saint Pierre
13885 Marseille Cedex
France

Mogensen CE
2 University Clinic of Internal
Medicine
Kommunehospitalet
DK-800 Aarhus C
Denmark

Moggi L
Istituto di Clinica Chirurgica
Generale
Università Degli Studi di Perugia
Policlinico Monteluce
06100 Perugia
Italy

Mulet Meliá J
Hospital Clínico Servicio de Cirugía
Cardiovascular
Villarroel 170
08036 Barcelona
Spain

Müller B
Schering AG
Postfach 650311
D-1000 Berlin
FRG

Nachbur B
Universitätsklinik für Thorax-,
Herz- u Gefäßchirurgie
Inselspital
CH-3009 Bern
Switzerland

* Natali J
66 Boulevard Malesherbes
75008 Paris
France

Norgren L
Department of Surgery
Lund University
S-22185 Lund
Sweden

Novo S
Viale delle Alpi 86
90144 Palermo
Italy

Ohlsen H
Department of Radiology
Karolinska Hospital
Box 60500
S-10401 Stockholm
Sweden

Pagnan A
Instituto di Medicina Clinica
Policlinico Universitario
Via Giustiniani 2
35100 Padova
Italy

Paoletti R
Institute of Pharmacological
Sciences
University of Milan
Via Balzaretti 9
20133 Milano
Italy

Pardy BJ
144 Harley Street
London W1N 1AH
UK

Partsch H
Dermatology Dept
Wilhelminenspital
Montleartstraße 37
A-1160 Vienna
Austria

Pedrini L
Cattedra di Chirurgia Vascolare
Policlinico S Orsola
Via Massarenti 9
40138 Bologna
Italy

Peters PE
Westfalische Wilhelms Universität
Albert-Schweitzer-Str. 33
4400 Münster
FRG

Poli A
Instituto Farmacologia
Via Balzaretti 9
20129 Milano
Italy

* Raff W
Schering AG
Postfach 650311
D-1000 Berlin
FRG

Ruckley CV
Vascular Surgery Unit
Edinburgh Royal Infirmary
Lauriston Place
Edinburgh EG3 9YW
UK

Schneider E
University Hospital
Medical Policlinic Angiology
Division
Rämistr 100
CH-8091 Zürich
Switzerland

Schoop W
Aggertalklinik
Gruhscheidt
D-5250 Engelskirchen
FRG

Schrör K
Institut für Pharmakologie
Heinrich-Heine-Universität
Düsseldorf
Moorenstraße 5
D-4000 Düsseldorf 1
FRG

Shaw JW
Dept of Diagnostic Radiology
Ninewells Hospital
Dundee DD1 9SY
UK

Sinzinger H
Atherosclerosis Research Group
Schwarzspanierstraße 17
A-1090 Vienna
Austria

Spraul M
Abteilung Ernährung u Stoffwechsel
MNR-Klinik
Universität Düsseldorf
Moorenstraße 5
D-4000 Düsseldorf
FRG

* Stock G
Schering AG
Postfach 650311
D-1000 Berlin
FRG

Strano A
Dipartimento di Medicina Interna
Universita "Tor Vergata"
Via di Vigna Stelluti 40
Rome
Italy

Taylor RS
Epsom District Hospital
Dorking Road
Epsom
Surrey KT18 7EG
UK

Tooke J
Royal Devon & Exeter Hospital
Barrack Road
Exeter
Devon EX2 5DW
UK

Trübestein G
Medizinische Poliklinik der
Universität
Wilhelmstraße 35–37
5300 Bonn
FRG

Van Urk H
University Hospital Rotterdam
40 Molewaterplein
3015 GD Rotterdam
The Netherlands

* Verstraete M
Center for Thrombosis & Vascular Research
University of Leuven
Herestraat 49
B-3000 Leuven
Belgium

Wolfe JN
St Mary's Hospital
Praed Street
London W2 1NY
UK

* The names of the Organising Committee are marked by an asterisk and correspondence relating to this document can be addressed to any one of them.

# Table of Contents

# Contributors

Professor Peter Bell
Department of Surgery, Clinical Sciences Building, Leicester Royal Infirmary, Leicester LE2 7LX, U.K.

Professor Vittorio Bertelé
Clinica Medica Generale, Universita di Milano, Ospedale L. Sacco, 20157 Milano, Italy

Professor Alfred Bollinger
Department of Internal Medicine, Medical Policlinic Angiology Division, University Hospital, CH-8091 Zurich, Switzerland

Professor Klaus Breddin
Centre of Internal Medicine, Division of Angiology, J.W. Goethe University, Theodor-Stern-Kai 7, D-6000 Frankfurt am Main 70, Federal Republic of Germany

Professor Maria Catalano
Clinica Medica Generale e Terapia Medica, Universita degli Studi di Milano, c/o Ospedale L. Sacco, via GB Grassi 74, 20157 Milano, Italy

Professor Chiara Cerletti
Istituto di Ricerche Farmacologiche, Mario Negri, Consorzio Mario Negri Sud, 66030 Santa Maria Imbaro, Italy

Mr. John Dormandy
Department of Vascular Surgery, St. James Wing, St. George's Hospital & Medical School, Blackshaw Road, London SW17 OQT, U.K.

Dr. Michael Edmonds
Diabetic Department, Kings College Hospital, Denmark Hill, London SE5 9RS, U.K.

Dr. Bert Eikelboom
Department of Surgery, St. Antonius Hospital, 3435 C M Niewegein, Netherlands

Professor Bengt Fagrell
Department of Medicine, Karolinska Hospital, S-10401 Stockholm, Sweden

Professor Jean-Noel Fiessinger
Service de Medecine Interne et de Pathologie Vasculaire, Hopital Broussais, 6 rue Didot, 75674 Paris Cedex 14, France

Dr. Giovanni de Gaetano
Istituto di Ricerche Farmalogiche Mario Negri, Consorzio Mario Negri Sud, 66030 Santa Maria Imbaro, Italy

Mr. Peter Harris
Vascular Surgery Unit, Ward 25, Broadgreen Hospital, Thomas Drive, Liverpool L14 3LB, U.K.

Professor Heinz Heidrich
Facharzt für Innere Medizin, Burggrafenstraße 1, D-1000 Berlin 30, Federal Republic of Germany

Dr. S. Rao Kadambari
Consultant Psychiatrist, St. George's Hospital & Medical School, London SW17 OQT, U.K.

Dr. Wolfgang Krings
Westfälische Wilhelms-Universität, Institut für Klinische Radiologie, Albert-Schweitzer-Str. 33, D-4400 Münster (Westf.), Federal Republic of Germany

Professor Wilhelm Krone
5th Floor, Room 500, University Hospital Eppendorf, 2000 Hamburg, Federal Republic of Germany

Dr. Gordon Lowe
Glasgow Royal Infirmary, Department of Medicine, 10 Alexandra Parade, Glasgow G31 2 ER, Scotland

Professor Felix Mahler
Angiologische Abteilung, Universitäts Hospital, CH-3010 Berne, Switzerland

Mr. Paul Moody
Vascular Surgery Unit, Broadgreen Hospital, Liverpool L14 3 LB, U.K.

Dr. Bernd Müller
Research Laboratories, Schering AG, D-1000 Berlin 65, Federal Republic of Germany

Dr. Dirk Müller-Wieland
University Hospital Eppendorf, 2000 Hamburg, Federal Republic of Germany

Professor Jean Natali
Department of Vascular Surgery, American Hospital of Paris, 63 Boulevard Victor Hugo, 92202 Neuilly Cedex, France

Professor Lars Norgren
Department of Surgery, Lund University, S-22185 Lund, Sweden

Professor Peter Peters
Westfälische Wilhelms Universität, Albert-Schweitzer-Str. 33, 4400 Münster, Federal Republic of Germany

Mr. Vaughan Ruckley
Vascular Surgery Unit, Edinburgh Royal Infirmary, Lauriston Place, Edinburgh EG3 9YW, Scotland

Dr. Peter Stirnemann
Angiologische Abteilung, Universitäts Hospital, CH-3010 Berne, Switzerland

Professor Günter Stock
Research Laboratories, Schering AG, D-1000 Berlin 65, Federal Republic of Germany

Professor Raymond Verhaeghe
Center for Thrombosis & Research, University of Leuven, Campus Gasthuisberg O & N, Herestraat 49, B-3000 Leuven, Belgium

Professor Marc Verstraete
Center for Thrombosis & Research, University of Leuven, Campus Gasthuisberg O & N, Herestraat 49, B-3000 Leuven, Belgium

# Chapter 1

## The Patient's Point of View – Psychological Concerns

S. Rao Kadambari



*"This is the great error of our day in the treatment of the human body, that physicians separate the soul from the body".*

PLATO

### 1.1 Introduction

The diagnosis of ischaemia, perhaps a further complication of a chronic debilitating illness, results in a further fall in self-esteem, loss of uniqueness and purpose, together with an increased sense of vulnerability and death. For these people, life seems more fragile and impermanent than it did before. "Why me?" voices concern for being punished for past misconduct, or that further harm will follow.

Recognition of imminent surgical treatments, possible loss of limb and much reduced life expectancy often produces a terrifying sense of helplessness, but at the same time there is typical disbelief and thoughts that "... this cannot really be happening to me". Consistent with such thoughts, many report a sense of detachment as though they were simply observers of the events taking place. Although this could be viewed as a defence against the threat of loss of limb, or death, it is also likely to be linked with incomprehension of the reality of the situation.

## 1.2 Pain

Most patients with critical leg ischaemia will have had a long experience of intermittent claudication. Age, obesity, smoking, diabetes mellitus, haemodynamic wear and tear all influence the origin and progression of the condition – and consequently the pain reaction. Patients may become less sociable, giving up hobbies, sports and other recreational activities. As arterial insufficiency progress, the claudication distance diminishes leading to eventual rest pain. This is so severe and relentless that it dominates the patient's whole life, both day and night. Ischaemic rest pain may progress to ischaemic ulceration. The patient's struggle continues for relief measures and he may obtain some help by hanging the foot and leg over the side of the bed, or putting it on a low chair beside the bed. Some patients sleep in a chair, or will get up several times during the night to pace the bedroom. They freely exhibit feelings of anger, anxiety, irritability, withdrawal or depression. Some will also resort to taking medication, using or misusing drugs, and this further complicates their mental health. Eventually, they avoid home- and employment-related responsibilities, along with the recreational activities already missed.

Each patient's communication of pain is determined by his past experience. Patients at similar stages of the disease vary in their response to pain; the elderly experience it less than the younger and pain thresholds tend to be lower in women than men [1, 2]. Other factors identified with persistent pain in cancer patients include disagreeable environment, anxiety, depression, poor general health, a long history of the disease and lack of confidence in the physician [3].

## 1.3 Denial

There is a high proportion of denial-like coping processes in patients with this severe, incapacitating illness which has positive adaptational consequences.

Although denial can be direct because of its unconscious status, it is more often than not inferred by indirect evidence, through behaviour which is said to mask, bolster or maintain denial. For example some patients experience euphoria and elation when ulceration is in progress with severe arterial insufficiency. Minimisation, disregard or delay in confronting real external problems, by means of various forms of attention deployment (for example booking a holiday), unless supported from outside, will not be successfully maintained for more than brief periods at a time. Without reinforcement from physicians, family, friends and others, denial within normal range probably could not be sustained.

Denial may take its toll, but it may also serve very important adaptive functions by conserving energy and postponing action. This has been observed in several studies, especially when reference is made to seriously ill patients such as those afflicted with cancer [4, 5] or myocardial infarction [6].

Stern et al. (1976) assessed the coping process following acute myocardial infarction and report "deniers" (representing 25% of the sample) were more generally optimistic, did very well returning to work, functioned better sexually and suffered less from post-coronary depression and anxiety [7]. This finding is consistent with Hackett et al.'s (1968) claim that denial of the danger of death may be associated with decreased mortality and better post-coronary adjustment in the coronary care unit [8].

## 1.4 Depressive Reaction

As denial diminishes, grief and depression emerge. Due to the nature of the disability, both physical and emotional, anxiety and sadness are to be expected as natural and appropriate. Furthermore, there is often some impairment of self-esteem [9]. The patient tends to mourn his loss of self. Among some patients, severely diminished self-esteem may manifest as a sense of helplessness, feeling that they are a burden to others and that they have nothing to offer [10]. They may resort to becoming uncommunicative or withdrawn, wish they were dead or vaguely think of suicide. If this idea develops into a specific plan, a specific time, circumstance, condition or method then there is considerable danger of actual suicide, and immediate intervention is mandatory. For some people the sense of loss of control over one's bodily functional abilities is countered by thoughts of the ultimate control: suicide.

## 1.5 Dissociation

For very few patients the limb pain, loss of function and ulcer is unbearable and they experience dissociation, where they describe an actual physicial separation of their intellectual and emotional selves from the body. They feel their cognitive selves to be located in another part of the room, in order to escape from the pain. This type of dissociation appears to be a health-saving coping mechanism, rather than a symptom of psychosis [11]. The experience leaves them with a sense of isolation from their previous identities, both physically and emotionally.

## 1.6 Death Wish

Some people have a passive desire for death to come and wash over them, carrying them away from pain and further surgery. This wish for death usually subsides with the stabilizing of body functions and gradual return of physical strength, but patients sometimes require a referral for more intensive counselling.

## 1.7 Limb Salvage Measures

Amputation is a serious undertaking; therefore reconstructive arterial surgery welcome. The operation is often rewarding for both the patient and the surgeon. However, the initial enthusiasm evaporates if the results are disappointing. Learning that repeated last resort surgical interventions to save the limb are not effective, and that the end result has to be amputation after all, can be difficult for many patients to accept, and demoralizing. Unsuccessfully completing a series of possible palliative treatments is extremely stressful and, to a major extent, jolt their patience and trust. The cost of these measures is discomfort for the patient, a waste of limited medical resources and further stress for care givers.

## 1.8 Amputation

How one comes to terms with the idea of amputation largely depends on the individual's estimate of the consequences of loss of limb, which not only depend on the patient's physical condition and results of earlier interventions, but also in some cases his economic and social background. Moreover, as long as his beliefs are different from the reality, he will not feel susceptible to the gangrene, and therefore will not submit to the amputation. However some patients, with self-esteem severely battered from recurrent failures, may passively accept and subject themselves to a long-delayed amputation in a state of emotionally neutral helplessness. Others may withdraw their consent and passively resort to suicide through their illness.

The threat may be complex; not just concerning immediate problems of pain, loss of limb and immobilisation, but also concerning the loss of control of events affecting the patient's life. Having no control, and not knowing how things will go in future, undermines personal security. How does the amputation affect independence, hobbies, social life, interpersonal and sexual relationships? It is the not knowing and not having control over the loss which triggers anxiety, depression, isolation and either rejection or acceptance for the loss of a limb. Age, race, sex, religion, culture, occupation, education, disposition, security and support all motivate patients in taking the major decision of an amputation.

## 1.9 Coping

Individual personality characteristics and coping techniques vary tremendously. Each person has unique hereditary and constitutional components, expressed in dispositions of temperament. These dispositions interact with specific familial environments, which reflect not only the broad cultural matrix of western civilisation and its ethos, but also narrowed subcultural characteristics. Each definition of self carries with it particular outlooks, attitudes and expectations for behaviour. Within this field of forces, every patient develops a typical style of perceiving, problem-solving, thinking and acting towards themselves and others.

Some patients strongly identify with "pain objects". They cope by touching, wearing and using specific objects. A "pain chair" gives great relief for some who believe they are able to endure pain and cope better with it. Some patients with a painful necrotic limb learn to cope by being able to concentrate enough and "... to imagine that the foot does not even belong to me – it hurts, it smells bad; I just decided not to think of it as mine".

Some patients gain respite from their distress by blocking out the awareness of threat and loss; they repress any thoughts that might excite emotional response. An inaccurate picture is thus presented; patients can be in considerable distress, but deny this to themselves and others. Other patients who experience severe pre-amputation distress together with feelings of helplessness, stoically accepting amputation, either delay recovery or may never achieve it, compared with patients who were characterized as having fighting spirit and deny their pain, ischaemia and amputation.

Despite these factors, a substantial number of patients make a satisfactory, if not heroic, adjustment with minimal distress. Patients who are allowed – and encouraged – to look, touch and help in dressing their own stumps progress well. Those who have not seen their stumps believe that the area is much worse than its actual appearance.

## 1.10 Conclusion

Most consultations are initiated by the patients for the relief of the pain and they require immediate reassurance. Doctors usually use the time in reaching an accurate diagnosis and planning the most appropriate "physical treatment". Consultation is a special type of encounter which Goffman has described as a focussed interaction in which both parties try to sustain a single focus of attention [12], based on the principle of holistic medicine that the illness exists in a whole person and not just in the organs. Consequently, therapeutic approaches to "cure" must, of necessity, include psychological parameters of illness. The majority of these patients will eventually depend upon various support systems such as their family, local or health authority institutions due to decreased physical function and emotional incapacitation. The family and carers should have the maximum support together with the opportunity to understand the illness and must also be brought in to assist in planning the treatment and future rehabilitation.

## References


1. Exton-Smith AM (1961) Terminal illness in the aged. Lancet II:305–308
2. Merskey H, Spear FC (1967) Pain: psychological and psychiatric aspects. Balilliere, Tindall & Cassel, London
3. Cole R (1965) The problem of pain in persistent cancer. Med J Aust 52:682
4. Aitken-Swan J, Easson EC (1959) Reactions of cancer patients on being told their diagnosis. Br Med J 1:779–783
5. Gilbertson VA, Wangensteen OH (1962) Should the doctor tell the patient that the disease is cancer? In: The physician and the total care of the cancer patient. American Cancer Society, New York, pp 80–85
6. Croog SH, Shapiro DC, Levine S (1971) Denial among male heart patients. Psychosom Med 33:385–397
7. Stern MJ, Pascale L, McLoone JB (1976) Psychological adaptations following an acute myocardial infarction. J Chronic Dis 29:513–526
8. Hackett TP, Cassem NH, Wishnie HA (1968) The coronary care unit: an appraisal of its psychoclogical hazards. N Engl J Med 279:1365–1370
9. Missel J (1978) Suicidal risks: the medical rehabilitation setting. Arch Phys Med Rehabil 59:351–376

10. Berbing E (1953) Mechanisms of depression. In: Greenacre P (ed) Affective disorders: psychoanalytic contribution to their study. New York International University Press Inc., pp 13–48
11. Fisher S, Cleveland SE (1958) The role of body image in the psychoneuroses and psychoses. Body image and personality. Van Nostrand, New York, pp 230–249
12. Goffman E (1961) Encounters. Bobbs-Merrill, Indianapolis

# Chapter 2

# Definition, Incidence and Epidemiology

Lars Norgren



Ischein haima, from the Greek, means to suppress blood. Ischaemic conditions in an extremity may imply anything from a slight claudication to an acute arrest of blood flow. Several expressions have been used and misused to describe a certain chronic limitation of the nutrition to an extremity, such as "Limb-threatening ischaemia", "severe ischaemia", "critical ischaemia" (Fig. 1).

Since the early 70's it has been accepted that surgical procedures are usually only justified for patients with more severe symptoms than claudication, especially if procedures below the groin are to be considered. Possibly the interpretation of "limb-threatening" has sometimes been extended to include relatively minor symptoms such as rest pain and fissures as ischaemic ulcers.

One of the problems which thereby emerges is the impossibility of comparing and interpreting results from different studies, or to ensure that patients in multicentre studies are included with similar criteria. This criticism is not primarily directed towards the subjective judgement of the patient, but more to the fact that objective measurements have not been used, or have been misinterpreted.

## 2.1 Definition

A strict definition of chronic critical limb ischaemia is necessary, not only for scientific reasons, but also for the evaluation of the result of treatment in this severely diseased group of patients. The definition could be very simple if all patients with a true limb-threatening condition went to amputation, if no radical improvement of blood flow could be achieved with surgery, interventional radiology or medical treatment. This is however not the case. Certain variations and fluctuations in the ischaemic stage are commonly present, and treatment of other conditions, such as a failing heart, may switch a critical to a noncritical leg ischaemia.

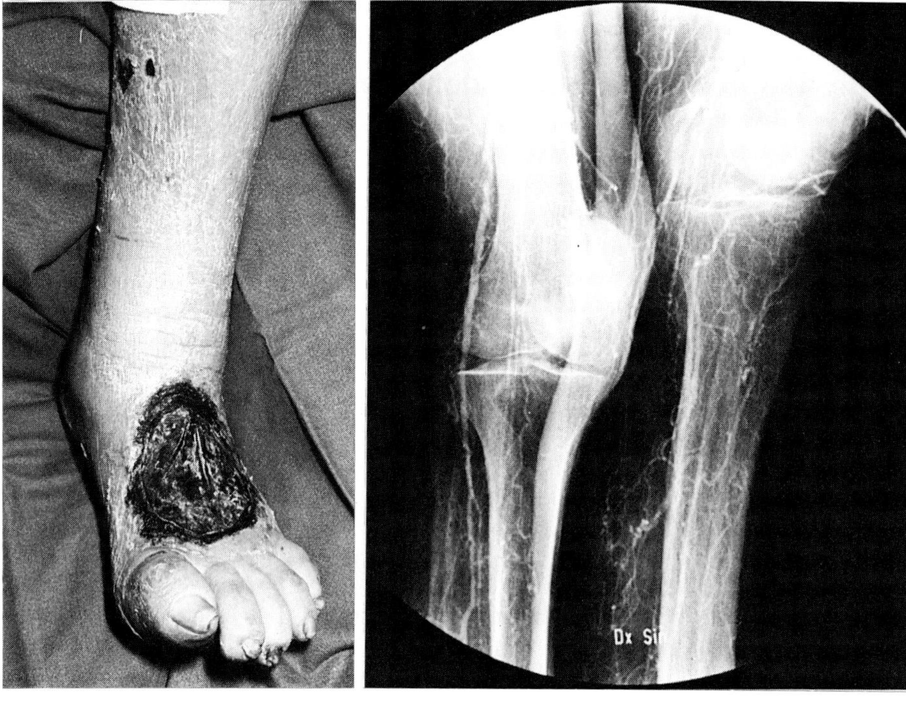


**Fig. 1 a and b.** The critical ischaemic limb with necrosis and ulceration (**a**). (**b**) Angiographic pattern from the same limb as (**a**). Note that only collaterals are visualized. On the opposite side (dx) severely arteriosclerotic main arteries are partly filled

In the vascular bible of the 40's, Peripheral Vascular Diseases by Allen, Barker and Hines [1], Ghormley stated that "most of the patients have spent months or years trying to avoid amputation", talking in favour of fluctuations in the condition at a time when reconstructive procedures were not yet available. From placebo controlled studies including critically ischaemic patients, it is evident that only about 50% of the patients in the placebo group are amputated within a year [2].

Efforts have been made to solve the problem and create definitions. The classification by Fontaine used especially in parts of Europe has defined two stages within which the term "critical ischaemia" may fit: stage III with rest pain and stage IV with ulceration or gangrene. Their correlation to ankle indices are shown in Table 1 [3].

During the International Vascular Symposium, London, 1981, a Working Party [4] devised definitions based on more objective criteria, and suggesting subgrouping in acute and chronic critical ischaemia. Considering chronic ischaemia only they proposed a lower limit of four weeks' symptoms. Measurements of ankle pressure were considered a prerequisite with $<40$ mm Hg as the limit, but if necrosis or gangrene was present the limit was increased to $<60$ mm Hg. An important statement was that diabetics and non-diabetics should not be mixed,

**Table 1.** Fontaine stages correlated with ankle pressure index [3]

| Stage | Symptoms/signs | Ankle pressure index (mean ± SD) |
|---|---|---|
| I | No clinical symptoms | 1.11 ± 0.10 |
| II | Intermittent claudication | 0.59 ± 0.15 |
| III | Ischemic rest pain | 0.26 ± 0.13 |
| IV | Ischemic ulcer, gangrene | 0.05 ± 0.08 |

giving rise to difficulties in presenting and interpreting results. This last statement needs careful consideration, since diabetics account for a considerable part of all critically ischaemic patients, and even if not overt diabetics, patients with pathological glucose load may create an intermediate population. A similar approach to the European Working Party was taken by an Ad Hoc Committee in USA [5].

The Joint Vascular Research Group [6] performed a prospective study to test these definitions, ending up with a slightly different terminology, using one out of two criteria: rest pain and ankle doppler pressure <40 mm Hg or rest pain with ulceration or gangrene. This classification is thus very close to the Fontaine grading. Scoring of vascular disease has been proposed as another possibility for uniform judgement [7].

With this background the European Working Group on Critical Limb Ischaemia started its work, with the aim of trying to reach consensus amongst different disciplines working with ischaemia, such as angiologists, vascular surgeons, basic scientists and radiologists.

The following general definitions were agreed [8]:

> "Critical ischaemia is defined by the following two criteria: Persistently recurring rest pain requiring regular analgesia for more than two weeks and/or ulceration or gangrene of the foot or toes, *plus* ankle systolic pressure < 50 mm Hg. R 2 A
>
> Calcification of the arteries in diabetes and other diseases makes measurement of the ankle pressure unreliable. Absent palpable pulses are sufficient for definition of critical limb ischaemia in diabetics, and patients with calcified arteries."

A more precise definition was recommended for published reports or for design and report of clinical trials. Besides the above definition, further evidence of ischaemia must be obtained by angiography or one of the following tests: toe-systolic blood pressure < 30 mm Hg; transcutaneous oxygen pressure of the ischaemic area < 10 mm Hg and which does not increase with inhalation of oxygen; absence of arterial pulsations in the big toe, measured with strain gauge or photoplethysmography after vasodilation; marked structural or functional changes of the skin capillaries in the affected area assessed by capillaroscopy. R 2 B

Evidently there is a need to link the Fontaine classification with the above definitions. This is possible by only a slight change of the Fontaine classification. Patients in Fontaine stage IV (ulceration or gangrene) have critical ischaemia, as well as some patients in stage III, who have an ankle pressure < 50 mm Hg. Stage III could thereby be subdivided into stage III A: rest pain plus ankle pressure above 50 mm Hg and stage III B: rest pain plus ankle pressure below 50 mm Hg. In that way stage III A is excluded from the definition critical limb ischaemia.

## 2.2 Incidence and Epidemiology

The true incidence of critical limb ischaemia with regard to the above definitions cannot be easily estimated. From other data, however, such as the incidence of amputation, there are possibilities to reach figures probably approximating the true incidence.

One way is to follow patients with peripheral arterial disease to see if any early signs of disease are predictors for future critical ischaemia. Rosenbloom et al. [9] followed 195 claudicating patients for 8 years, finding that as much as 41% deteriorated to rest pain or tissue loss. Fifty per cent of the patients had died during the follow up period. An initial decrease of the ankle-brachial index after exercise was found significantly associated with a subsequent development of critical ischaemia. The level of the disease was however not found that reliable. By contrast, Jonasson and Ringqvist presented data [10] suggesting that multilevel disease implied a lower 6-year survival than that of patients with a single stenosis.

Källerö [11] found a correlation between morbidity and mortality in coronary heart disease and localization of the atherosclerotic disease to the lower leg trifurcation.

In the extensive literature survey by Dormandy et al. [12] it was found that even patients with claudication, but no critical ischaemia, had a more than doubled mortality rate within five years, compared to the general population. From this data it was not possible to extrapolate which proportion of the patients would deteriorate to critical ischaemia. Two of the studies in the survey, the Basle study and the Framingham study [13, 14] showed however very similar figures for subsequent amputation rates in claudicants, between 1.6–1.8%. Irrespective of the definition of critical limb ischaemia the majority of all studies on the natural history of ischaemic patients present a five year mortality rate of about 50%. The amputation rate may on the other hand differ according to which form of treatment the actual study is presenting.

Recently a Swedish study [15] was presented comprising 167 patients with critical ischaemia, where vascular surgery or interventional methods for various reasons were not performed. These patients were followed for five years. The criterion of critical ischemia was only rest pain. Thirty per cent of the patients were diabetics; the mortality rate within five years was 50% for non-diabetic atherosclerotic patients and 60% for diabetics. Fifty per cent of those surviving five years were amputated. Interestingly, there was no significant difference between amputation rate for those with necrosis and those without. The results are very close to findings from Denmark in the sixties [16].

The incidence of amputations in Sweden was 17 per 100000 in the fifties and is now around 50 per 100000. The increase since 1910 is shown in Fig. 2 from the

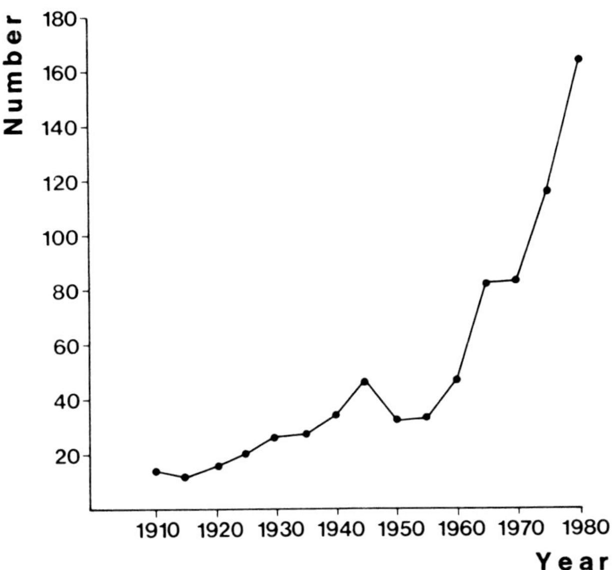


**Fig. 2.** The increase in amputations since 1910. (From Liedberg 1983)

thesis of Liedberg [17]. In his study the proportion of diabetics was found to be 37%. According to the DHSS [18] the aetiology of 5582 leg amputations performed in 1986 in England, Wales and Northern Ireland was 63.9% in non-diabetic vascular disease and 83.9% if diabetics are included.

Tracy et al. [19] 1982 found that for the USA the number of amputations performed annually almost matched the number of arterial reconstructions.

From the studies referred to and from other data it can be estimated that the prevalence of peripheral arterial disease in the whole population is 5% in men aged over 50 years but only less than 10% of those will probably deteriorate to critical ischaemia. For diabetics the incidence is higher; probably there is a five times higher risk for diabetics of developing critical ischaemia.

From the number of major amputations, it can be estimated that the incidence of critical limb ischaemia is approximately 500–1000 per million population per year. Such a figure takes into consideration that a considerable number of patients die before they come to amputation and that the majority of the patients benefit from vascular surgery or other revascularisation procedures.

It is well known that the incidence of thromboangitis obliterans is low in Europe, but nevertheless a proportion of the critically ischaemic patients will suffer from that disease. The population seems to have a different natural history than the atherosclerotic group. A Japanese study [20] found that the risk of amputation was less than half of that for a comparable group of patients with atherosclerosis. Furthermore the life expectancy for the thromboangitis obliterans group approached that of the general population.

## 2.3 Prognosis

The life expectancy of critically ischaemic patients undergoing reconstructive vascular procedures differs from those who need an amputation. Two studies [21, 22] have shown a better survival rate for those reconstructed, but evidently there may have been a difference in the severity of the disease in these two groups.

With new reopening procedures, which may also be used in less fit patients, such as PTA, laser- and mechanical angioplasties and thrombolysis, the future will show whether limb saving even in such a situation will also become life saving.

Even if in general terms the fate of an amputee is worse than of a limb salvaged patient, it is important to discuss when revascularization should be performed. Without doubt there are patients whose prognosis is worsened due to a delayed amputation, after a failed revascularization or failed medical treatment. For the individual patient it is therefore always important to evaluate both the chance of saving life and saving limbs.

Another important objective is today the cost/benefit discussion [23] which however may not be interpreted that the cost is more important than other factors.

Summarizing available data, it seems that in diabetic patients with critical ischaemia about 20% undergo PTA and 15% reconstructive vascular surgery. A mixed population with critical ischaemia is treated with reconstructive vascular procedures in 60% and 20% undergo amputation. After one year 20% have died and 25% have had a major amputation.

## References


1. Ghormley RK (1946) Amputation in occlusive arterial diseases. In: Allen, Barker, Hines (eds) Peripheral vascular diseases. WB Saunders, Philadelphia, pp 783–800
2. Norgren L (for the Study Group) (1988) Iloprost versus placebo in patients with ischemic ulcers. A Scandinavian-Polish multicenter study. Presented at the Angiodyn, Toulouse, France
3. Yao ST (1970) Hemodynamic studies in peripheral arterial disease. Br J Surg 57:761–766
4. Bell PRF, Charlesworth D, DePalma RG et al. (1982) The definition of critical ischaemia of a limb. Br J Surg 69:2
5. Ad Hoc Committee on Reporting Standards (1986) Suggested standards for reports dealing with lower extremity ischemia. J Vasc Surg 4:80–94
6. Wolfe JHN (1986) Defining the outcome of critical ischaemia. A one year prospective study. Br J Surg 73:321
7. Walden R, Modan M, Bass A et al. (1989) Scoring of vascular disease in the lower extremities. J Cardiovasc Surg 30:210–215
8. European Consensus Document on Critical Limb Ischaemia. Dormandy J (ed) (1989) Springer, Berlin Heidelberg New York
9. Rosenbloom MS, Flanigan DP, Schuler JJ et al. (1988) Risk factors affecting the natural history of intermittent claudication. Arch Surg 123:867–870
10. Jonasson T, Ringqvist I (1985) Mortality and morbidity in patients with intermittent claudication in relation to the location of the occlusive atherosclerosis in the leg. Angiology 36(5):310–314
11. Källerö KS, Bergqvist D, Cederholm C et al. (1984) Arteriosclerosis in popliteal artery trifurcation as a predictor for myocardial infarction after arterial reconstructive operations. SGO 159:133–138

12. Dormandy J, Mahir M, Ascady G et al. (1989) Fate of the patients with chronic leg ischaemia. J Cardiovasc Surg 30:50–57
13. Widmer LK, Biland L, DaSilva A (1985) Risk profile and occlusive peripheral artery disease. In: Proceedings of the 13th International congress of Angiology. Athens
14. Kannel WB, McGee DL (1985) Update on some epidemiological features of intermittent claudication. J Amer Geriatrics Soc 33:13–18
15. Bohlin T, Aldman A, Gustavsson PO et al. (1988) Hur går det för patienter med viloischemi som ej opereras? Läkartidningen (Swedish) 85:2398–2399
16. Mathiesen FR, Larsen EE (1966) The natural history of leg ischemia measured by plethysmography. J Cardiovasc Surg 36:498–500
17. Liedberg E, Persson BM (1983) Increased incidence of lower limb amputation for arterial occlusive disease. Acta Orth Scand 54:230–234
18. DHSS. Statistics and Research division. Amputation statistics for England, Wales and N. Ireland 1976–1986
19. Tracy GD, Lord RSA, Hill DA et al. (1982) Management of ischemia of the foot beyond arterial reconstruction. SGO 155:377–379
20. Ohta T, Shionoya S (1988) Fate of the ischemic limb in Buerger's disease. Br J Surg 75:259–262
21. Eichhoff JH (1988) Amputation and arterial reconstruction for severe ischemia of the lower limbs. Ugeskr Laege 75:259–262
22. Myers KA, King RB, Scott DF et al. (1978) Surgical treatment of the severely ischemic leg. I. Survival rates. Br J Surg 65:460–464
23. Gupta SK, Veith FJ, Ascer E et al. (1988) Cost factors in limb threatening ischemia due to infrainguinal arteriosclerosis. Eur J Vasc Surg 2:151–154

## *Commentary*

*Maria Catalano*

The continual readjustments to the definition and consequently the epidemiology of critical limb ischaemia are closely linked to developments in therapeutic possibilities. The definition of this condition has in fact been repeatedly updated at various meetings of experts. In addition to Fontaine stage IV, a third stage has been considered in which pain would persist for four (in the previous definitions) or two (present definition) weeks (API $<50$ mm Hg). This variation is obviously related to criteria for therapeutic intervention. The incidence of critical limb ischaemia has also been modified by the efficacy of previous therapeutic intervention in the subjects in stage II and stage III a.

However, a definition of the disease is still a fundamental prerequisite to establishing an epidemiological database and provide objective measurements of the efficacy of therapeutic interventions, which cannot be obtained in small groups of non homogeneous patients.

It is thus difficult at present to provide epidemiological data on a disease entity variously defined in the available studies. In the absence of data, alternative means must be used which, indirectly, estimate the direct incidence and prevalence of this disease. The following approaches, each with its own intrinsic errors and limitations, are possible:

*(1) Prevalence of peripheral arterial disease in the general population and the proportion who ultimately develop critical limb ischaemia*

The generally accepted prevalence of peripheral vascular disease (PVD) is around 1 or 1.5%. In the major European studies it has varied from 0.9 to 6.9% of the population in the age group 50–60 years [1]. This data, however, is based only on the presence of symptoms of claudication and may be a gross underestimate of the prevalence of peripheral vascular disease. This is demonstrated in various studies in which a prevalence of 20% was revealed when the history and clinical findings were considered together, whereas the prevalence rose to 27.7% when instrumental diagnostic investigations were also taken into account [2]. Although there is much uncertainty about the true prevalence of peripheral vascular disease in the general population, it is widely agreed that 20–30% of patients with vascular disease will have significant progression of their disease within 10 years and 3 to 6% will ultimately require an amputation.

Prospective studies have reported unhomogeneous data on amputation after follow-up of five to 11 years. The major studies show the influence of age, other associated risk factors and initial severity of arterial disease on the prognosis. Widmer's data exemplify this: at 11 years he observes 19% of amputations in elderly patients versus 2.4% in younger subjects with less severe arterial disease and 0.5% in controls.

*(2) Prevalence and incidence of PVD and its progression in diabetics*

Diabetes is well known to be one of the major vascular risk factors and affects from 2–5% of the european population with high differences between countries, with a further 10–15% not diagnosed according to WHO data. The prevalence of PVD in diabetics varies with age and duration of the disease, and is more frequent in type II diabetes. In a WHO study performed in 14 centres in 13 countries on diabetics aged between 35 and 55 years, the prevalence of PVD was 3.5% in the men and 2.6% in the women. 1.4% presented with claudication and 1.6% had been amputated (2% in the men and 1.3% in the women) [4]. Also in this case the consideration of claudication and amputation alone led to an underestimation. According to other studies, the prevalence of PVD between 50 and 70 years varies from 8% to 22% in diabetics versus 3% in the controls. Furthermore, the incidence of PVD in diabetics was 14% at two years [5], 15% at 10 years and 45% at 20 years [6]. Progression of PVD is formidable: at two years 87% of diabetics worsening of the disease showed as assessed by Doppler pressure measurements [5].

Analysis of specific data on amputations in diabetics shows that amputation is 15 times more frequent in diabetics than in controls, with the proportion of amputation (major and minor) in diabetics being 3.7%, 31.9% and 64.4% in subjects under 45, 45–64 and over 65 respectively [7]. Two studies found that the risk of contralateral amputation is 53% at four years [8, 9]. Data from US show a prevalence of amputations in diabetics of 14 per 1000 and annual incidence of 40000 amputations in a total of 5500000 diabetics (plus those not diagnosed) [10]. In a prospective study on a population at high risk for diabetes followed for 12 years the incidence of first amputation (minor and major) was 2.2 per 1000 per year in the population analyzed, 0.1 in 1000 per year in the non diabetics and 10.4 in 1000 per year in the diabetics, with a maximum value of 28.4% in the subjects over 65 [11].

*(3) Official data on the prevalence and incidence of amputations*

From the data reported in the Consensus Document the incidence of major amputation varies from 120 to 300 cases per million per year. The response is greatly influenced by the accuracy and efficiency of the national or regional data collection and analysis services. Furthermore, these represent failures in treating critical limb ischaemia and should not be confused with the latter.

*(4) Cardiovascular mortality*

The association between ischaemic heart disease, cerebrovascular disease and peripheral arterial disease is important and it has been observed in 30 to 90% of cases, depending on the stage of the disease. A review of the literature indicates that PVD mortality is 20–30% at five years, 60% at 10 years and 75% at 15 years [13]. Also mortality in diabetics is greatly influenced by an association with PVD: 4% of diabetics die at two years versus 22% of diabetics with arterial disease of the lower extremities. The severity of arterial disease has a strong effect on survival of the patients. In a study that evaluated the weight of various factors on cardiovascular mortality the expected life lost at 12 years was 20% for patients with claudication and 44% for patients with advanced ischaemia [14]. Lastly, in amputated subjects the reported survival is 50–70% at five years, whereas it falls to 64% already at one year when the patients are also diabetic.

To conclude, efforts to define critical limb ischaemia should be accompanied by efforts to centralize epidemiological data and the results of the various therapeutic choices in order to establish a common study programme.

## *References*

1. Reunanen A, Tukkunen H, Aromaa A (1982) Prevalence of intermittent claudication and its effect on mortality. Acta Med Scand 211:249–256
2. Criqui MH, Fronek A, Connors EB et al. (1985) The prevalence of peripheral arterial disease in a defined population. Circulation 3:510–515
3. Blombery PA (1987) Intermittent claudication. An update on management. Drugs 34:404–410
4. Diabetes Drafting Group (1985) Prevalence of small vessel and large vessel disease in diabetic patients from 14 centers. The World Health Organisation Multinational Study of Vascular Disease in Diabetics. Diabetologia 28:615–640
5. Beach KW, Bedford GR, Bergelin RO et al. (1988) Progression of lower extremity arterial occlusive disease in type II diabetes mellitus. 11:464–472
6. Melton LJ, Macken KM, Palumbo J et al. (1980) Incidence and prevalence of clinical peripheral vascular disease in a population based cohort of diabetic patients. Diabetes Care 3:650–654
7. Billd DE, Selby JV, Sinnock P et al. (1989) Lower extremity amputation in people with diabetes. Epidemiology and prevention. Diabetes Care 12:24–31
8. Most RS, Sinnock P (1983) The epidemiology of lower extremity amputations in diabetic individuals. Diabetes Care 6:87–91
9. Silbert S (1952) Amputation of the lower extremity in diabetes mellitus. Diabetes 1:297–299
10. Mazze RS, Sinnock P, Deeb L et al. (1985) An epidemiological model for diabetes mellitus in the United States: five major complications. Diabetes Research and Clinical Practice 1:185–191
11. Nelson RG, Gohdes DM, Everhart JE et al. (1988) Lower extremity amputations in NIDDM. 12-Yr follow-up study in Pima indians. Diabetes Care 11:8–16
12. Callam MJ, Harper DR, Dale JJ et al. (1987) Arterial disease in chronic leg ulceration: an underestimated hazard? Lothian and Forth Valley leg ulcer study Br Med J 294:929–931
13. Coffman JD (1986) Intermittent claudication: not so benign. Am Heart J November: 1127–1128
14. Lassila (1986) Peripheral arterial disease – natural outcome. Acta Med Scand 220:292–299

# Chapter 3

# Pathophysiology of Critical Leg Ischaemia

Gordon Lowe



## 3.1 Introduction

Critical leg ischaemia has been defined previously in this volume as foot ischaemia which is of sufficient severity to cause either pain at rest or skin necrosis (ulceration or gangrene). It is likely that rest pain arises from nerve endings in ischaemic skin, stimulated by the end-products of hypoxic metabolism. However it has been suggested that ischaemic neuropathy may also cause foot pain. In contrast, skin necrosis is commonly painless in diabetics, due to anaesthesia from diabetic neuropathy (see Chapter 10). A low ankle pressure (less than 50 mm Hg), or absent ankle pulses in diabetics, is also included in the definition. This criterion confines the syndrome to the common problem of ischaemia produced primarily by occlusive disease of the large proximal arteries supplying the lower limb, and excludes ischaemia produced by primary microvascular occlusion (e.g. microthromboembolism).

Traditionally, critical leg ischaemia has been viewed as a "plumbing problem". Bypass grafting of an occluded major artery (or more recently, disobliteration of the blocked artery by angioplasty, catheter aspiration or throm-

**Table 1.** Summary of pathophysiological factors in the ischaemic lower limb

| Site | Haemodynamics | Cells and chemistry |
|---|---|---|
| Heart | Cardiac embolism | |
| | Cardiac output | |
| | Hydrostatic pressure | |
| Arteries | Low shear stresses → atherosclerosis | Lipids, lipid peroxides |
| | Plaque rupture → thrombosis | Endothelial disturbance (VWF, t-PA, PAI-1, $PGI_2$, EDRF, EDCF, EDGF) |
| | → Increased proximal resistance | Fibrin formation/fibrinolysis |
| | Decreased blood pressure ← | Platelet and leucocyte activation and adhesion |
| | ↓ Decreased blood flow | Shear release of ADP from RBC |
| | → Collateral formation | |
| Arterioles | → Vasodilatation, vasomotor paralysis | |
| | (vasoconstriction in some areas?) | |
| Capillaries | → Flow maldistribution (reduced functional density) | Endothelial cell swelling and disturbance (VWF, t-PA, PAI-1. $PGI_2$, EDRF, EDCF, EDGF) |
| | → Altered vasomotion (small flux-motion waves) | Platelet microaggregates, microthrombosis |
| | → Increased permeability oedema, Capillary collapse → | Leucocyte plugging |
| | | RBC plugging |
| Venules, veins | Deep vein thrombosis | RBC aggregation |
| | Venular thrombosis | |
| | Increased venous resistance | Leucocyte margination |

bolytic enzymes) has been the main focus of surgical and medical therapy. However in recent years there has been increasing interest in the microcirculatory disturbance which follows large vessel occlusion, as well as in the haemorheological, haemostatic and inflammatory consequences (Table 1). There is increasing evidence of interactions between these changes in the small vessels and the blood. During the workshop on pathophysiology, which was part of the Consensus process, an initial attempt was made to illustrate these interactions and their potential to promote ischaemia at the level of the microcirculation in the foot.

These efforts were stimulated partly by early reports of the clinical successes of medical treatments of critical leg ischaemia, including analogues of endogenous mediators such as prostacyclin.

This chapter reviews the macrocirculatory, microcirculatory, biochemical and haematological changes which may promote critical leg ischaemia. Haemodynamic factors are considered first, and biochemical and haematological factors second (Table 1). However this is an artificial distinction, because it is likely that there are interactions between haemodynamics and both cellular and chemical factors at all levels of the ischaemic limb (Table 1).

## 3.2 Haemodynamics of Critical Leg Ischaemia

### 3.2.1 The Heart

Confronted with a patient with critical leg ischaemia, the clinician should consider three possible pathogenetic contributions of the heart: its potential as a source of emboli to the lower limb; its output of blood to the lower limb; and its position relative to the lower limb which determines the hydrostatic pressure of the arterial blood column (Table 1).

Acute limb ischaemia due to a large embolus detaching from within the heart is a well-recognized syndrome, frequently cured by urgent embolectomy. Cardiac emboli may also contribute to subacute critical leg ischaemia, and should be suspected in patients with deep vein thrombosis ("paradoxical" embolism through a patent foramen ovale), atrial fibrillation (atrial thrombi), heart valve disease or prosthesis (atrial or valve thrombi; vegetations from endocarditis), or recent myocardial infarction (mural thrombi). Suitable cardiac investigations are outlined in the Consensus Document. Intracardiac thrombus can be visualized by cardiac ultrasound, and anticoagulant therapy should be considered in such patients to prevent further embolism.

Reduction in cardiac output may result from dysrhythmias, from decreased myocardial contractility, or from obstruction (e.g. severe aortic stenosis, pulmonary embolism, cardiac tamponade). Rarely, low-output heart failure may cause peripheral gangrene even in the absence of occlusive peripheral arterial disease [1]. More commonly, a reduction in cardiac output by disease or drugs may precipitate critical leg ischaemia in patients with occlusive peripheral arterial disease. For example, the onset of atrial fibrillation reduces cardiac output by about 10 percent: such a fall in perfusion pressure may tip the balance towards critical ischaemia in an elderly patient with multiple level arterial occlusions in the lower limb. Hence the haemodynamic effects of atrial fibrillation should be considered as well as its embolic potential. Myocardial infarction or pulmonary embolism can have similar haemodynamic results, as well as embolic potential. Beta-adrenergic blocking drugs, often prescribed to patients with peripheral arterial disease for treatment of concomitant hypertension or angina, can precipitate critical ischaemia, possibly due to reduction in cardiac output as well as decrease in peripheral blood flow [2]. Over-zealous use of other antihypertensive drugs may also decrease peripheral perfusion to a critical level.

The Consensus Document therefore suggests that clinicians should routinely
R 3 assess cardiac status, including chest X-ray and electrocardiography, in investigating patients with critical limb ischaemia; and should treat heart failure
R 6,7 and dysrhythmias, avoiding hypotension and beta-adrenergic blockers.

Dependency of the feet increases hydrostatic pressure, which in patients with critical leg ischaemia distends the peripheral vascular bed, reducing vascular resistance and increasing blood flow (see Section 3.3). However, dependency also promotes leg oedema which may reduce nutritive capillary flow. Hence the Consensus Document suggests that patients with critical leg ischaemia and skin necrosis should have the affected limb placed in the lowest possible position
R 9 without oedema formation.

### 3.2.2 The Arteries

Atherosclerosis of the lower abdominal aorta and its branches to the lower limbs is a primary cause of lower limb ischaemia, both intermittent claudication and critical leg ischaemia. Significant arterial disease of the lower limbs is usually accompanied by disease of the coronary and carotid arteries [3]. This fact probably accounts for the high risk of heart attacks and stroke, which between them kill over 80 percent of patients with lower limb ischaemia [4] (see Chapter 2).

Risk factors for peripheral arterial disease, which may operate partly through atherogenesis, include smoking, triglyceride, and (less certainly) blood pressure, cholesterol and glucose intolerance [4]. Smoking and diabetes have been predictive of amputation for critical limb ischaemia in some prospective studies [4], and again their atherogenic effects may be relevant. As in other parts of the arterial tree, atherosclerotic lesions tend to occur at sites of flow disturbance, which suggests that haemodynamic factors are important [3] such as low shear stresses [5].

Critical leg ischaemia occurs when arterial stenoses increase proximal limb vascular resistance so severely that foot blood flow fails to meet the nutritive requirements of the resting limb. Chronic ischaemia may be compensated at two levels: (a) the development of collateral channels; and (b) reduction of peripheral limb vascular resistance by arteriolar vasodilatation (see Section 3.2.3). The onset of critical leg ischaemia implies the inadequacy of these compensations, and often results from the presence of multiple arterial occlusions at several levels, in critical collateral vessels, or in end-arteries [6]. The ankle systolic arterial pressure
R 2 falls (a pressure less than 50 mm Hg is suggested in the definition of critical leg ischaemia in the Consensus document), as does the ankle/arm systolic pressure index [7] and also the toe blood pressure. Because the pressure drop increases as blood moves distally through successive vascular beds, the clinical features of critical limb ischaemia (rest pain, ulceration and gangrene) usually start in the toes, and progressively involve the feet and lower leg. Blood flow to the feet and toes is considerably less per volume of tissue than blood flow to the hands and fingers, which may explain in part the more frequent occurrence of ischaemic necrosis in the toes than the fingers in the presence of comparable degrees of major vessel occlusion [6].

There is increasing evidence that plaque rupture and arterial thrombosis play a role in atherogenesis, as well as in precipitation of critical ischaemia and infarction [8]. Rupture of an atherosclerotic plaque, possibly initiated by high shear stresses, can initiate haemorrhage within the plaque, thus exposing blood platelets to tissue factors as well as to pro-aggregatory adenosine diphosphate (ADP) released from red blood cells. This platelet activation may trigger either (a) intra-plaque thrombus, with subsequent healing of the lesion by endothelialisation to produce a larger plaque; (b) non-occlusive luminal thrombus; or (c) occlusive luminal thrombus. Any of these events could precipitate critical ischaemia in the leg by increasing proximal limb arterial resistance to a critical level. The history of onset of critical leg ischaemia is frequently acute or subacute, consistent with such an acute arterial lesion. Correspondingly, fresh thrombus is often demonstrated at surgery for critical limb ischaemia, or by successful catheter or chemical thrombolysis. The recent demonstration of elevated levels of plasma cross-linked fibrin degradation products in patients with critical limb ischaemia compared to patients with intermittent claudication [9] is also consistent with a thrombotic precipitation of critical leg ischaemia. Occasionally, arterial thrombosis may follow arterial damage during diagnostic or therapeutic arterial puncture or catheterisation procedures.

In theory, critical increases in proximal limb arterial resistance could arise from arterial spasm, as well as atherosclerosis and thrombosis. Such spasm has been demonstrated angiographically in the coronary arteries, and in the cerebral arteries following subarachnoid haemorrhage. Spasm has also been observed during diagnostic or therapeutic catheterisation of lower limb arteries, especially in younger subjects with relatively muscular arteries. However there is little direct evidence for a role for spasm in precipitation of critical leg ischaemia in the absence of obvious causes of mechanical or chemical arterial injury.

### 3.2.3 The Microcirculation

In recent years there has been increasing interest in the microcirculation and its abnormalities in critical leg ischaemia, due partly to the development of new measurement techniques. The use of such techniques in investigation of patients is also considered in Chapter 4.

The ankle and/or toe systolic blood pressures are useful in evaluating the total arterial circulation to the distal lower limb [6, 7, 10–12]. Segmental blood pressure measurements at different levels of the leg can also supply information regarding the levels and severity of arterial occlusions [11]. In patients with intermittent claudication, the Doppler ankle/arm pressure index was also the most useful variable for predicting total cardiovascular events in the placebo group of a large clinical trial: the PACK Study [13], presumably as a sensitive index of generalised atherosclerosis. However there is a wide overlap between ankle blood pressure (or pressure index) or toe blood pressure when patients with critical leg ischaemia are compared to patients who have peripheral arterial disease but without critical ischaemia [6, 7, 11, 12, 14–17]. Some patients with zero toe blood pressure in the horizontal position do not develop critical leg ischaemia [12, 15] while other patients with relatively high toe blood pressure do develop critical leg ischaemia [12, 16, 18]. These findings suggest the importance of microvascular blood flow in pathogenesis of critical leg ischaemia.

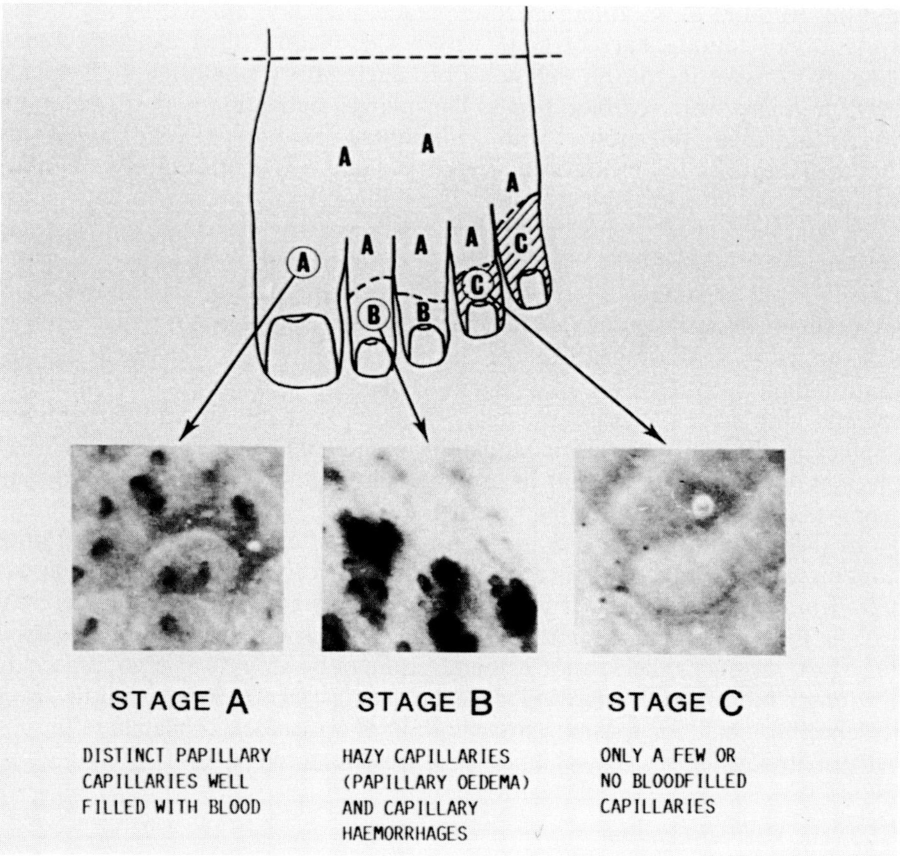


**Fig. 1.** Three stages of structural change in nutritional skin capillaries, observed by vital capillary microscopy in different regions of an ischaemic foot. A graphic illustration of microvascular flow maldistribution within the foot. Note increased capillary permeability (oedema) and capillary disruption (haemorrhages) in Stage B, and the lack of capillary perfusion in Stage C. Reproduced with permission from Fagrell and Lundberg [17]

One microvascular compensation which tends to maintain nutritional blood flow in the presence of proximal arterial obstruction is arteriolar vasodilatation, which lowers peripheral limb vascular resistance [6]. At an ambient temperature of 20° C, toe blood flow averages about 11 ml/100 ml tissue/minute, but rises to 21 ml/100 ml/min under the influence of a vasodilator drug [30]. In critical limb ischaemia, the arterioles may become maximally vasodilated and insensitive to normal vasoconstrictor stimuli – "vasomotor paralysis" [19]. Such vasodilatation may be mediated largely by vasoactive metabolites released from ischaemic tissue. Ischaemic rest pain typically develops at night, partly due to minimum flow in the circadian rhythm [20], and partly due to the horizontal posture. Elevation of the feet reduces hydrostatic pressure, and with autoregulation paralysed, reduction in transmural pressure causes collapse of capillaries, venules and veins.

"Pallor on elevation" is then seen in the foot skin. When the feet are dependent, the increase in hydrostatic pressure distends the passive, paralysed vascular bed, reducing peripheral resistance and increasing flow. On examination, the feet become suffused with a characteristic red-purple colour ("rubor on dependency"). Patients with nocturnal rest pain commonly learn to relieve pain by hanging their feet out of the bed, walking about, or sleeping in a chair [6].

Some patients with ischaemic rest pain or ulceration have, paradoxically, *higher total foot blood flow* in the ischaemic foot compared to the normal one [19]. This presumably arises from maximal vasodilatation in response to neighbouring areas of severe ischaemia [19]. The ultimate cause of ischaemic skin lesions is therefore presumably *maldistribution* of microcirculatory blood flow in the skin of the foot, rather than reduced total foot blood flow. About 90 percent of distal foot blood flow normally passes through non-nutritional, subpapillary, thermoregulatory vascular beds which bypass the nutritional, papillary skin capillaries through arterio-venous anastomoses [21]. It is therefore necessary to study nutritive microcirculatory blood flow in the different regions of the foot skin. This can be achieved by either capillary microscopy [12] or fluorescein angiography [22].

*Capillary microscopy* has shown a variety of abnormalities in nutritive skin capillaries in areas of the foot which develop ischaemic lesions [12, 23]. The simplest, three-stage classification is shown in Fig. 1 [17]. Stage A shows distinct papillary capillaries well-filled with blood. Stage B shows hazy capillaries (papillary oedema) and capillary haemorrhages. Stage C shows only a few or no blood-filled capillaries.

In a comparative prospective study, Fagrell and Lundberg showed that Stage C changes were 87 percent sensitive and 95 percent specific for the development of skin necrosis; and that the addition of capillary microscopy therefore improved the predictive value of toe blood pressure measurement (Fig. 2) [17]. These results demonstrate the importance of disturbed nutritive blood flow in the pathogenesis of ischaemic skin necrosis, rather than decreased digital perfusion pressure *per se*.

*Fluorescein angiography,* videomicroscopy and videodensitometry can be used to follow the appearance, distribution in capillary areas, transcapillary diffusion and interstitial distribution of intravenously-injected sodium fluorescein. Abnormalities observed in critical leg ischaemia include delayed inflow (fluorescein appearance time over 55 seconds), and increased capillary permeability in ischaemic areas of skin [22]. Studies combining fluorescein dye uptake with simultaneous measurement of *transcutaneous oxygen tension* ($tcPO_2$) [24] have shown that in critical leg ischaemia there is a normal *anatomical* capillary density (31–42/$mm^2$), but a reduced *functional* capillary density due to a pronounced *spatial heterogeneity of perfusion*. This maldistribution of microcirculatory perfusion is caused partly by total stasis in some capillaries, partly by reduced flow velocity in others, and partly by the presence of "plasmatic capillaries" which have an extremely reduced local haematocrit and which may comprise up to 30 percent of the capillary bed in such patients. The significantly delayed appearance of fluorescein in these abnormally-perfused capillaries was associated with greatly-reduced $tcPO_2$ (0–8 mm Hg). $TcPO_2$ measurements *per se* have shown decreased

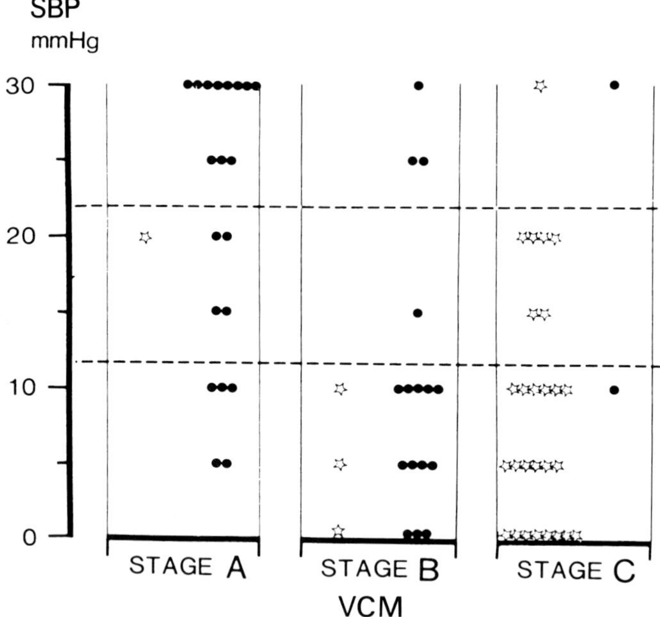


**Fig. 2.** The relationship between the systolic toe blood pressure (SBP) and the worst capillary stage found at vital capillary microscopy in the toes and forefoot (VCM) in 69 patients with critical leg ischaemia. (☆) patients developing skin necrosis; (●) patients not developing skin necrosis. The superior sensitivity and specificity of VCM over SBP in prediction of skin necrosis is evident. Reproduced with permission from Fagrell and Lundberg [17]

basal values (as well as delayed increases following arterial occlusion) in patients with peripheral arterial disease and critical leg ischaemia, and have been used to predict the probability of ulcer healing or of primary wound healing after amputation [25, 26].

*Laser-Doppler flux measurement* [27] has also been used in microcirculatory studies of critical leg ischaemia. Skin perfusion is studied to a penetration depth of approximately 1 mm, and hence both nutritive and non-nutritive (thermoregulatory) flow are measured. In critical leg ischaemia, *alterations in vasomotion* have been observed by this technique [27, 28]. Vasomotion describes the rhythmic distribution of flow to the capillaries. In critical leg ischaemia there may be a reduction in low-frequency motion waves (3–12/min) and the appearance of small flux-motion waves with a higher frequency ($21 \pm 4$/min) which are not found in health. This ischaemia-related vasomotion pattern disappears after successful percutaneous transluminal angioplasty [29].

Several potential causes of maldistribution of microcirculatory blood flow have been suggested. These include microthrombosis [30]; spasm of precapillary arterioles; collapse of the precapillary arterioles because of a low transmural pressure [10]; oedema [12]; endothelial cell swelling; abnormalities in vasomotion; or rheological occlusions [5] – which include red cell aggregates [31], rigid red cells [32], platelet aggregates [33] and rigid or adhesive white cells [34]. These processes are obviously potentially interactive. Some biochemical and haematological factors relevant to these processes are considered in Section 3.3.

### 3.2.4 The Veins

Decreased capillary perfusion in critical leg ischaemia may sometimes reflect venous obstruction as well as arterial inflow deficiency. *Cardiac failure* results in decreased systemic venous return and leg oedema, both of which reduce perfusion pressure in addition to the concomitant decrease in systemic arterial outflow (Section 3.2.1). *Deep vein thrombosis* also decreases venous return and increases oedema in the lower limb, sometimes to an extent which decreases capillary perfusion and threatens skin viability (venous gangrene or *phlegmasia caerulea dolens*). Urgent thrombolytic therapy or thrombectomy may be required for such critical leg ischaemia. Deep vein thrombosis may be a commoner contributor to critical leg ischaemia than is generally realised. Pulmonary embolism is common in patients undergoing amputation for critical leg ischaemia: predisposing factors include advanced age, decreased leg blood flow and foot dependency, all of which encourage venous stasis. Anticoagulant drugs may have a place in prevention of venous thromboembolism in these patients. R 30

*Diffuse thrombosis of small skin veins* may also cause critical leg ischaemia in purpura fulminans, coumarin-induced skin necrosis, and severe protein C deficiency. The latter usually occurs in homozygous neonates; however the author has observed it following coumarin overdose in an adult heterozygous for protein C deficiency. In this case the critical leg ischaemia responded to intravenous infusions of heparin and fresh frozen plasma (protein C replacement) and decompression of the foot skin by application of leeches followed by fasciotomy.

## 3.3 Biochemical and Haematological Factors in Critical Leg Ischaemia

Several biochemical and haematological factors have been reported to be abnormal in patients with critical and/or non-critical lower limb ischaemia [35]. However it is not usually possible to establish from systemic arm vein measurements their relationships to generalised arterial disease, lower limb arterial disease, microcirculatory disturbances, or associated risk factors. Few studies have performed measurements in lower limb venous blood as well as arm vein blood in order to study their relevance to lower limb ischaemia. Equally there are few prospective studies to determine their prognostic significance for critical ischaemia in patients with non-critical lower limb ischaemia, or for survival of the patient and/or his limb in patients with critical leg ischaemia. Such studies are required in order to further assess the significance of biochemical and haematological variables in critical leg ischaemia. Several of these variables are also known to be abnormal in diabetes, and these abnormalities (which are discussed in Chapter 10) may be relevant to the increased propensity of diabetics to critical leg ischaemia.

### 3.3.1 Lipids and Lipid Peroxides

Serum cholesterol is a risk factor for premature coronary artery disease: however its relationship to peripheral arterial disease is much poorer [4]. Serum triglyceride may show a stronger relationship to peripheral arterial disease, however prospective studies are required [4]. Lipid peroxides, formed by the peroxidation of unsaturated fatty acids, are present in aortic atherosclerotic lesions [62] and show increased plasma levels in peripheral arterial disease [36, 37]. In the latter study, plasma lipid peroxide levels correlated with plasma triglyceride levels, but not with the presence of critical leg ischaemia [37]. Low density lipoproteins can be oxidised by free radicals generated by endothelial cells, monocytes and neutrophils; they may in turn promote endothelial cell injury, uncontrolled lipid uptake by macrophages, decreased endothelial synthesis of prostacyclin (prostaglandin $I_2$, $PGI_2$) and thrombosis [37]. Further studies are required to assess the significance of lipids and lipid peroxides in peripheral arterial disease; however at present their rôle appears to be in the earlier stages of atherogenesis rather than in the late stage of critical ischaemia.

### 3.3.2 Endothelium

Endothelial disturbance is one possible initiating factor for both thrombosis in limb arteries, and for capillary leakage and oedema, platelet aggregation and microthrombosis, and leucocyte adhesion in the ischaemic microcirculation. Endothelial cell products which might be potential markers of endothelial disturbance (Table 1) include von Willebrand factor (vWF); tissue-type plasminogen activator (t-PA) and its endothelium-derived major inhibitor (plasminogen activator inhibitor type 1, PAI-1); prostacyclin ($PGI_2$); endothelium-derived relaxing factor (EDRF); endothelium-derived constricting factor (EDCF); and endothelium-derived growth factor (EDGF). It is noteworthy that major risk factors for critical limb ischaemia such as cigarette-smoking and diabetes are associated with abnormalities of several of these endothelial markers (vWF, t-PA and $PGI_2$), supporting the hypothesis that endothelial disturbance may be one link between these risk factors and limb ischaemia.

The endothelium plays a key role in maintaining vascular patency. Firstly, it removes from the circulation and/or degrades active mediators of thrombosis (e.g. ADP, adenosine triphosphate (ATP), serotonin (5-hydroxy-tryptamine, 5-HT) and thrombin). Secondly, it secretes prostacyclin and EDRF which prevent vasoconstriction by arterial and arteriolar smooth muscle cells (SMC) and which prevent platelet activation. Thirdly, it secretes t-PA which prevents excessive fibrin deposition and microthrombosis.

On the other hand, the endothelium also plays an active role in haemostasis. Following endothelial injury, release of vWF promotes platelet adhesion to subendothelium; release of EDCF may initiate vasoconstriction; release of PAI-1 may protect fibrin haemostatic plugs from premature dissolution by t-PA; and release of EDGF may promote cell proliferation as part of subsequent tissue repair processes.

*Von Willebrand Factor*

Von Willebrand factor is a high molecular weight multimer, released from vascular endothelium, which promotes platelet adhesion to subendothelium. Deficiency (von Willebrand's disease) results in defective primary haemostasis and a clinical bleeding disorder. Elevated plasma vWF levels have been reported in peripheral arterial disease [38] but their prognostic significance and relevance to critical leg ischaemia are not yet known.

*Tissue-type Plasminogen Activator and its Inhibition*

There are a few reports in the literature of impaired fibrinolysis in peripheral arterial disease, which may favour atherogenesis, arterial thrombosis, and microthrombosis [35, 39, 40]. It is likely that such defective fibrinolysis reflects decreased production of t-PA by endothelium, and/or increased production of PAI-1 (which may also be produced by platelets and hepatocytes). There are methodological problems in measurement of these two interacting proteins, and further studies are required to assess their pathogenetic significance in peripheral arterial disease, as well as their relationships to risk factors such as smoking and diabetes. A variety of agents have been shown to stimulate endogenous fibrinolysis, e.g. anabolic steroids which reduce elevated PAI-1 levels. However, as yet, there are only anecdotal reports of their use in peripheral arterial disease [40].

*Prostacyclin*

Prostacyclin ($PGI_2$) is a potent vasodilator and inhibitor of platelet aggregation, which is released from arterial endothelium by mechanical injury or by interactions with platelets or leucocytes. While a rôle for defective $PGI_2$ production in atherogenesis has been postulated [39], patients with extensive atherosclerosis have *increased* $PGI_2$ production, possibly due to increased platelet-vascular interactions [41]. $PGI_2$ production is difficult to measure and the prognostic significance of $PGI_2$ disturbances is unknown. The rôle of prostanoids in treatment of critical limb ischaemia is considered in Chapter 9.

*Endothelium-Derived Relaxant Factor*

EDRF may protect arteries and arterioles against vasoconstrictor influences, e.g. leukotrienes released from activated leucocytes [42]. The generation of superoxide radicals by leucocytes may result in breakdown of EDRF and hence loss of vasodilatation [43]. However, disturbances in EDRF have yet to be demonstrated in patients with leg ischaemia. Similar constraints apply to the postulated rôles of EDCF and EDGF in peripheral arterial disease.

### 3.3.3 Platelets

A variety of alterations in platelet behaviour have been reported in patients with peripheral arterial disease. These include increased plasma levels of platelet release products such as beta-thromboglobulin and serotonin (5-HT); increased plasma levels of platelet prostanoid pathway products such as thromboxane $B_2$; shortened platelet survival time; shortened skin bleeding time; decreased platelet count; increased mean platelet volume; and increased platelet adhesiveness and aggregability *in vitro* [33, 35, 41, 44]. These abnormalities may reflect either intrinsic changes in platelets; or extrinsic factors such as high shear stresses at arterial stenoses, increased haematocrit levels, or increased plasma fibrinogen levels [33]. Forconi et al. reported increased beta-thromboglobulin levels in femoral vein blood drawn from patients with intermittent claudication following ischaemic lower limb exercise, suggesting the further possibility of local platelet activation under ischaemic conditions [45]. However, the prognostic significance of these changes and their relationship to critical leg ischaemia is unknown. Increased platelet aggregate formation is also observed in nonvascular illnesses such as chest infections [33].

A contribution of platelets to proximal atherosclerosis in the lower limb is suggested by the study of Hess et al. who showed that platelet inhibition by aspirin and dipyridamole delayed progression of angiographically-documented lesions [46]. This effect was more marked in smokers or hypertensives than in non-smokers or normotensives. However, this study provided no data of clinical interest, for example progression of symptoms or need for surgery. Indeed, there is little evidence that anti-platelet agents are of clinical value in intermittent claudication, although some have suggested that longterm aspirin be prescribed, extrapolating from meta-analyses suggesting benefit to patients with coronary or cerebral arterial disease [47].

The potential contribution of platelet microaggregates to microvascular occlusion in critical leg ischaemia is illustrated by the rare condition of thrombocythaemia, in which there are increased numbers of circulating platelets, increased platelet aggregability *in vitro,* and microvascular ischaemia even in the absence of large vessel occlusive disease [16, 35]. Such microvascular ischaemia responds to treatment with aspirin with or without dipyridamole [16, 35]. However the efficacy of these anti-platelet drugs in patients with the much commoner type of critical leg ischaemia due to primary large vessel occlusion is not established.

Intravenous or intra-arterial infusion of prostanoids has been reported as beneficial in treatment of critical leg ischaemia [47] (see Chapter 9). Possible mechanisms include reduction in platelet deposition on atherosclerotic lesions (demonstrated by Sinzinger et al. in studies of radio-labelled platelets); and reduction in microcirculatory occlusions by platelet aggregates. Defibrination with ancrod also reduces platelet aggregate formation [33] which may be relevant to its effect in increasing nutritive skin blood flow in ischaemic feet [48].

### 3.3.4 Fibrin Formation

As previously discussed, arterial thrombosis and microthrombi may play important rôles in critical leg ischaemia. Such thrombi are composed of fibrin as well as platelets, and the clinical success of thrombolytic therapy in critical leg ischaemia (see Chapter 8) illustrates the importance of this fibrin component. A variety of disturbances in blood coagulation which may favour fibrin formation have been described in peripheral arterial disease, including elevated levels of fibrinogen and factor VIII, shortened clotting times, and decreased levels of the coagulation inhibitor antithrombin III [35]. Elevated fibrinogen levels increase plasma and blood viscosity as well as favouring fibrin formation (Section 3.3.6). Decreased fibrinolysis in patients with peripheral arterial disease may also favour fibrin deposition (Section 3.3.2). Until recently, there was little evidence that fibrin formation was increased in peripheral arterial disease, as measured by increased plasma levels of fibrin degradation products [35]. However, we have recently shown that patients with intermittent claudication have higher levels of cross-linked fibrin degradation products, measured by a sensitive immunoassay, compared to controls; and that patients with critical leg ischaemia have further increases, due possibly to arterial and/or microcirculatory fibrin deposition [9]. Prospective studies of cross-linked fibrin degradation products and other markers of activated coagulation are currently in progress in patients with peripheral arterial disease.

There is little evidence that anticoagulants are effective in treatment of critical leg ischaemia, apart from their previously-mentioned rôle in prevention of venous thromboembolism. However they may be of general benefit in patients R 30
with chronic peripheral arterial disease, as shown by increased patient survival in a randomised controlled trial of patients after femoropopliteal vein bypass surgery [49].

### 3.3.5 Leucocytes

There is increasing evidence that white blood cells may contribute to arterial disease via atherogenesis, thrombosis and ischaemia [5, 50]. In hyperlipidaemic models of atherosclerosis, deposition of monocytes and neutrophils on arterial endothelium is one of the earliest observed events [51]. Monocytes can transform into macrophages and secrete growth factors as well as interleukin-1, which induces the adherence of further neutrophils and monocytes, and which may stimulate hepatocyte synthesis of fibrinogen as well as release of neutrophils from bone marrow. Activated leucocytes produce proteolytic enzymes, leukotrienes, superoxide anions, and platelet activating factor (PAF) which may produce endothelial cell and tissue damage and platelet activation: these processes may enhance atherogenesis and thrombosis in arteries, as well as ischaemia and microthrombosis in the microcirculation. The breakdown of EDRF by leucocyte-derived superoxide radicals has already been mentioned (Section 3.3.2). Not only can activated leucocytes activate platelets [52]: activated platelets can also activate neutrophil leucocytes [53].

Patients with intermittent claudication have higher leucocyte counts than controls, possibly as part of a generalised reactive process including increased plasma fibrinogen and viscosity [54]. However claudicants did not have increased leucocyte activation as shown by filterability through micropore filters [54]. On the other hand, patients with critical limb ischaemia did have leucocyte activation as shown by filtration studies [34]: this was more marked in blood sampled from the ischaemic limb veins than in systemic arm vein blood, and was normalised following reconstructive surgery [34]. Similar findings have been shown in patients with acute cerebral infarction as well as in acute chest infection, suggesting that leucocyte activation may be a nonspecific response to tissue injury whether vascular or nonvascular [55]. Nevertheless, there are a variety of possible mechanisms by which activated leucocytes may promote ischaemia in the presence of proximal arterial occlusion [5, 50].

Animal studies have suggested that in ischaemia in various organs, the impaction of leucocytes in the microcirculation causes "no-reflow" following restoration of arterial inflow [5, 50]. This may initially reflect plugging of nutritive capillaries by leucocytes, whose rigid nuclei render them three orders of magnitude less deformable in capillaries than erythrocytes. Activation by local ischaemic conditions may then increase the adhesive force between impacted leucocytes and capillary endothelium, contributing to the "no-reflow" phenomenon. Such increased adhesiveness of activated leucocytes may also increase their adhesion to venules in ischaemic organs, which will also increase microvascular flow resistance and promote leucocyte emigration into ischaemic tissues. The activation products of leucocytes may then promote endothelial disruption, increased microvascular permeability, cytolysis, platelet aggregation, and vasospasm. All such processes may contribute to critical leg ischaemia.

In man, the marked effects of increased numbers of immature, rigid leucocytes on nutritive flow in skin capillaries in leukaemic subjects have been described by Tooke and Milligan [63], illustrating the potential of leucocytes to promote microvascular obstruction. As yet, there are no prospective studies of leucocytes or their activation products in peripheral arterial disease, although the white cell count was found to be adversely predictive of reocclusion of distal bypass reconstruction [13]. Furthermore, the stabilising effects of prostanoids on leucocytes may be relevant to their therapeutic effects in critical leg ischaemia (Chapter 9).

### 3.3.6 Blood Rheology

In the normal limb, the intrinsic flow properties of blood (rheology) probably have little influence on blood flow. The viscosity (flow resistance) of bulk blood is low, due to shear-induced deformation of flexible red cells in parallel with flow streamlines. In the arterioles, a fall in dynamic haematocrit (the Fåhraeus effect) results in a further fall in blood viscosity (the Fåhraeus-Lindqvist effect). In the nutritive capillaries (diameter 3–15 μm) blood flow is again facilitated by the ready deformation of normal erythrocytes (resting diameter 7–8 μm), lubricated by low-viscosity plasma. In the leg veins, blood viscosity increases due to haemoconcentration (especially in the dependent foot) and to red cell aggregation as flow rates and hence shear rates fall; however this is of little consequence in healthy persons [5].

Blood viscosity increases in peripheral arterial disease, due to increases in both haematocrit and plasma fibrinogen levels: these changes result in part from the effects of cigarette smoking [35, 36, 56]. The increases are greater at low shear rates, due to red cell aggregation. In critical leg ischaemia, a further increase in fibrinogen (already raised in smokers and diabetics, and further increased by ischaemic necrosis and infection) results in further increases in plasma viscosity and erythrocyte aggregation.

The potential of blood viscosity increases to promote atherogenesis may be greater in the low-shear areas where lesions tend to occur, due to local viscosity increases under low-shear conditions. Increased blood viscosity may also increase shear forces on endothelial and blood cells as blood flows through critical arterial stenoses, promoting shear activation of leucocytes and platelets. Shear activation of platelets may be direct, or indirect via shear-induced release of ADP from red cells, or via shear-induced release of leucocyte activation products. The low shear areas distal to such stenoses may again favour local increases in blood viscosity, favouring interaction of activated platelets, leucocytes and clotting factors with the vascular wall as they mix in vortices. Thrombogenesis may well be favoured in such "*in vivo* aggregometers" [5].

In critical leg ischaemia, reduction in perfusion pressure also increases blood viscosity in the distal microcirculation. Decreases in blood flow rates decrease the Fåhraeus and Fåhraeus-Lindqvist effects, resulting in increases in haematocrit and blood viscosity, which may be exacerbated by haemoconcentration due to increased capillary permeability, vasodilatation and the dependent position of the foot ("rubor on dependency"). Increased blood viscosity is favoured not only by increased haematocrit, but also by increased fibrinogen levels (see above) and decreases in shear rate which promote red cell aggregation and loss of red cell deformation. Increased red cell aggregation also promotes white cell adhesion in venules: the Fåhraeus-Vejlens effect [5].

The filterability of blood through micropore filters which mimic nutritive capillaries (pore diameter 5 μm) also decreases in peripheral arterial disease, with greater increases in critical leg ischaemia compared to intermittent claudication [32]. This is probably due to leucocytosis and increased plasma viscosity in claudicants, because the filtration of erythrocyte and leucocyte suspensions in buffer is normal in such patients [54]. However, the greater impairment of filterability in critical leg ischaemia may reflect also leucocyte activation [34] as discussed in Section 3.3.5. Ischaemic conditions (e.g. leg exercise in claudicants) further reduce blood filterability and increase blood viscosity, probably due to the effects of lactic acidosis, activation of platelets and leucocytes, hyperosmolarity, and calcium influx into blood cells [45]. The ability of erythrocytes and leucocytes to deform and pass through nutritive capillaries is decreased in ischaemic limbs *in vivo*, due to the fall in perfusion pressure as well as the changes described above.

The contribution of rheological factors to critical leg ischaemia is suggested by the adverse prognostic significance of blood viscosity and fibrinogen levels in intermittent claudication [57]; the adverse prognostic significance of haemoglobin levels in healing of amputations for critical leg ischaemia [13, 58]; and the adverse prognostic significance of fibrinogen in claudicants [59] and in critical leg ischaemia [60].

Haemodilution may be successful in some patients with critical leg ischaemia [61] but awaits evaluation in large randomised trials. Meanwhile, haemodilution is recommended for consideration in patients with haematocrits over 50 percent in the Consensus Document, if it persists after rehydration and cessation of
smoking. Reduction in plasma fibrinogen and hence in plasma and blood vis- R 32

cosity following defibrination with ancrod may increase nutritive blood flow in ischaemic foot skin [48] but again such therapy awaits evaluation of efficacy in large controlled trials. The same constraint applies to other drugs with claimed haemorheological effects.

## 3.4 The Concept of Breakdown of the Microvascular Flow Regulating and Microvascular Defence Systems in Critical Leg Ischaemia

One result of the pathophysiological workshop on critical leg ischaemia in the Consensus process was an initial attempt to synthesise some of the possible biochemical and haematological factors promoting critical leg ischaemia into an overall concept of breakdown of body systems.

The *microvascular flow regulating system (MFRS)* was conceived as a system maintaining normal microvascular flow (Fig. 3).

Normal vasomotion ensures regular, periodic perfusion of nutritive capillary networks in foot skin, resulting in maintenance of healthy tissue. The endothelium maintains vascular patency by uptake and/or degradation of activating mediators; by the secretion of $PGI_2$ and EDRF which prevent platelet aggregation and vasoconstriction by smooth muscle cells (SMC); and by secretion of t-PA which prevents excessive fibrin deposition. Circulating red blood cells, white blood cells and platelets pass readily through nutritive capillaries in their resting, non-adherent, non-secretory states.

The *microvascular defence system (MDS)* comprises defences against both traumatic blood loss (i.e. haemostasis) and against infection (i.e. inflammation) (Fig. 4). In haemostasis, endothelial damage results in vasoconstriction (partly mediated by EDCF, and partly mediated by platelet release of 5-HT and secretion of thromboxane $A_2$, $TXA_2$) and release of vWF which promotes platelet adhesion. Shear damage to red blood cells also releases ADP which promotes platelet aggregation. Activation of platelets results in exposure of adhesion recep-

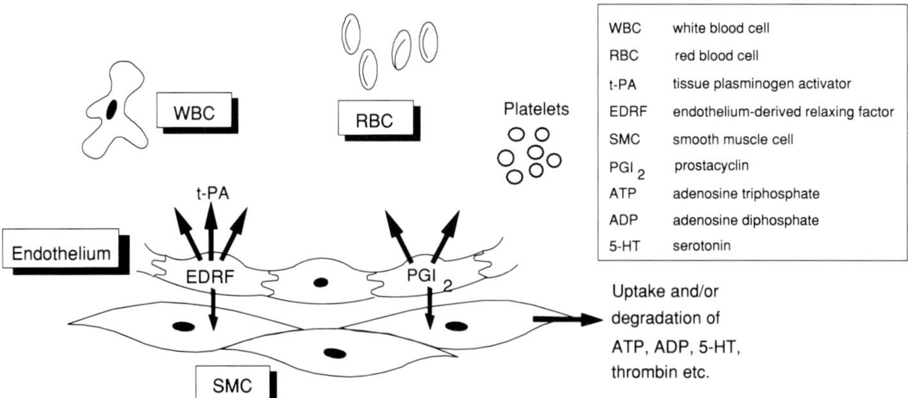


**Fig. 3.** The Microvascular Flow Regulating System (MFRS). The blood cells (WBC, RBC, platelets) are under physiological conditions in a non-adhering, non-secretory state. For description see text

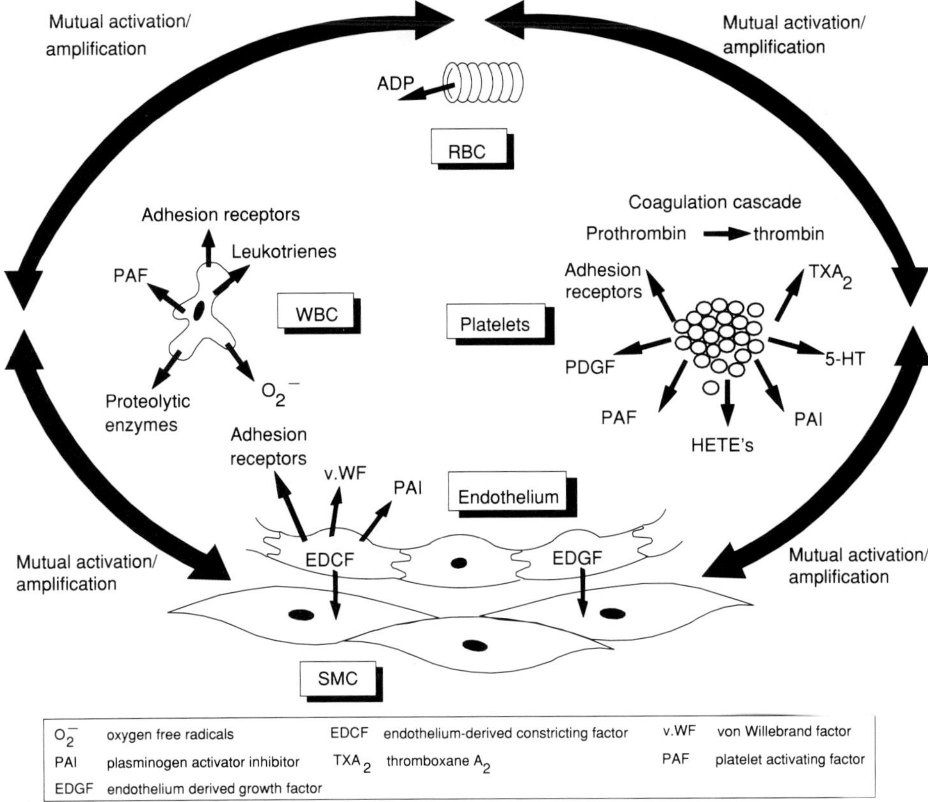


**Fig. 4.** Activation of the Microvascular Defence System (MDS). For description see text

tors (e.g. glycoprotein Ib which interacts with vWF promoting adhesion to subendothelium); release of 5-HT and formation of $TXA_2$ which promote vasoconstriction and platelet aggregation; and activation of the coagulation system which generates thrombin, which promotes both further platelet aggregation and fibrin formation, which reinforces the initial platelet haemostatic plug. Both platelets and endothelial cells release PAI-1 (which prevents breakdown of fibrin) and also growth factors (EDGF and platelet-derived growth factors, PDGF) which may play a role in subsequent tissue repair. Activation of leucocytes (e.g. by platelet release of HETE's) may also play a role in subsequent tissue repair following arrest of bleeding.

In the inflammatory response to *infection,* activation of neutrophils results in expression of adhesion receptors and secretion of proteolytic enzymes, leukotrienes and superoxide anions. Adhesion receptors are also exposed on endothelial cells, promoting leucocyte-endothelial interactions. The toxic effects of leucocyte products destroy both micro-organisms and (inevitably) some tissue cells, prior to subsequent tissue repair processes.

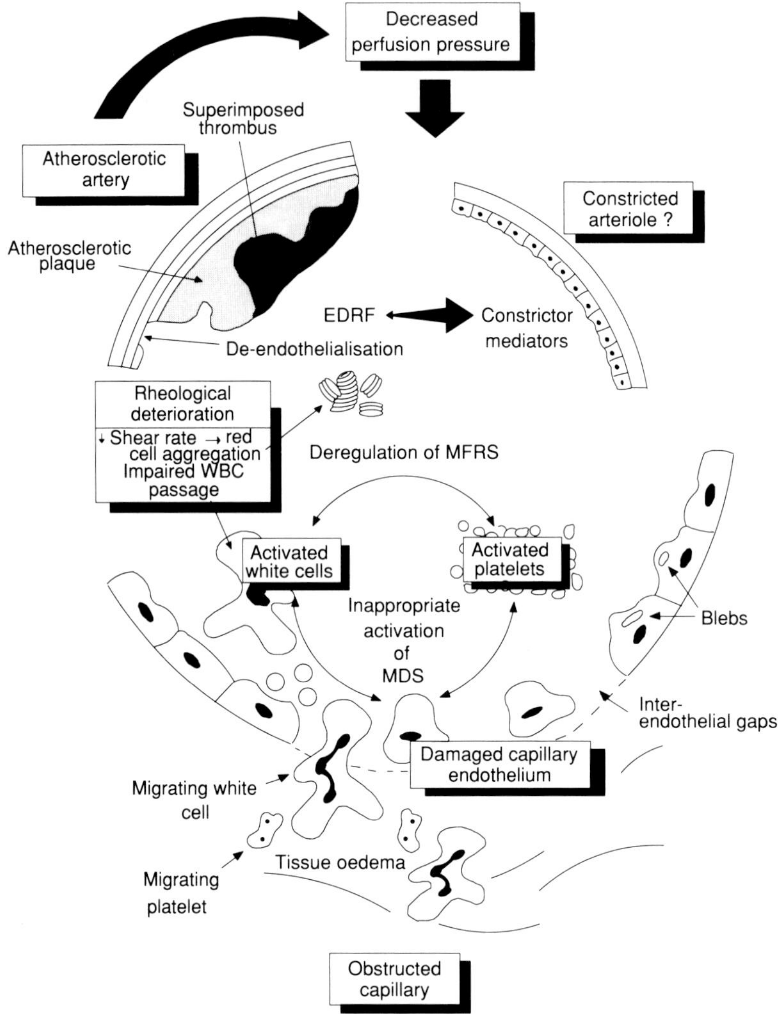


**Fig. 5.** Processes leading to critical limb ischaemia, in the arteries (upper left quadrant), arterioles (upper right quadrant) and microcirculation (lower half). For description see text

In both haemostasis and the inflammatory response to infection, there are many potential pathways for mutual activation and amplification of these interactions between endothelial cells and blood cells: these have been omitted from Figs. 3 and 4 for clarity.

In *critical leg ischaemia,* it is suggested that inappropriate activation of the MDS and breakdown of the MFRS may promote ischaemia, by enhancing both proximal arterial occlusion and microcirculatory flow disturbance (Fig. 5).

In *limb arteries,* activation of the MDS may result at a proximal atherosclerotic plaque following endothelial disruption and activation of platelets and leucocytes (e.g. by high shear forces). Such processes may initiate thrombosis on

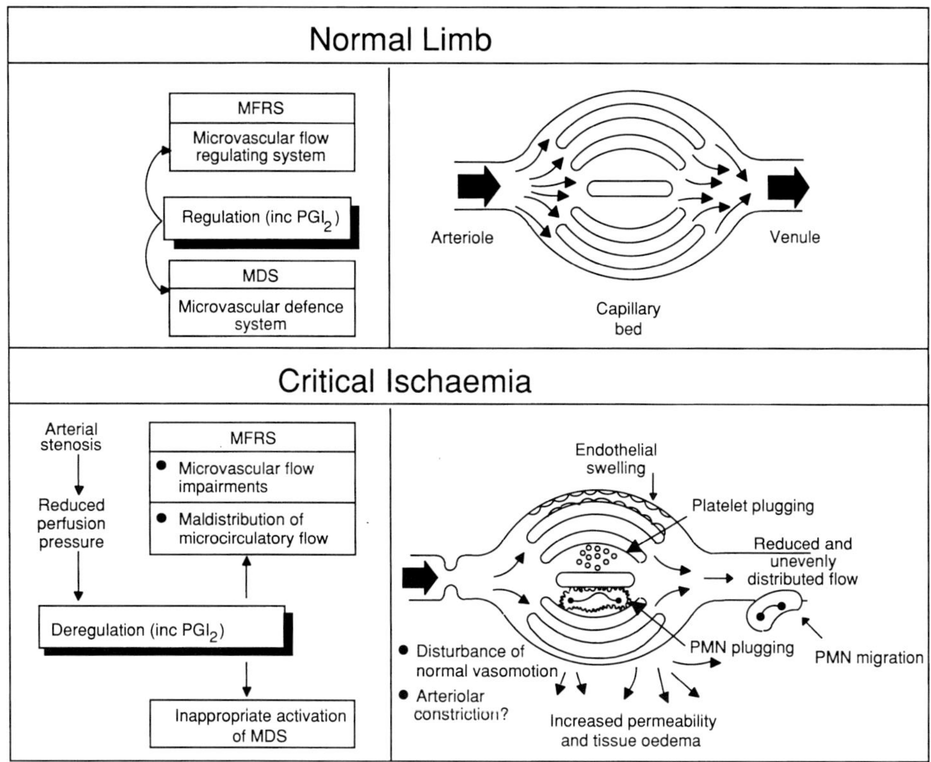


**Fig. 6.** Some causes of microcirculatory flow maldistribution in critical leg ischaemia. For description see text

the ulcerated arterial plaque, which critically reduces perfusion pressure and hence reduces blood flow in the distal limb (see upper left quadrant of Fig. 5).

In the distal *arterioles,* activation of the MDS may shift the balance of vasoregulatory mediators away from vasodilatation (e.g. generation of superoxide radicals by activated leucocytes results in breakdown of EDRF and therefore loss of vasodilatation) and towards vasoconstriction (e.g. release of 5-HT and formation of $TXA_2$ by activated platelets). Arteriolar vasoconstriction may then be one factor causing maldistribution of microcirculatory flow (see upper right quadrant of Fig. 5).

In the distal *microcirculation,* a variety of pathological processes may interact to further promote maldistribution of blood flow (see lower half of Fig. 5). Reduction in perfusion pressure lowers shear rates, which results in red cell aggregation and decreased passage of rigid leucocytes and erythrocytes through nutritive capillaries. Derangement of the MFRS occurs, with relative deficiency of $PGI_2$ and EDRF, and excess of vasoconstrictor mediators. Activation of the MDS results in interacting activations of leucocytes and platelets, which favour capillary obstruction by leucocytes and platelet aggregates, as well as endothelial cell damage (visible microscopically as blebs, interendothelial cell gaps, and endothelial cell swelling which may cause capillary obstruction). Increased capillary permeability and the activation products of migrating leucocytes promote tissue oedema, which is a further cause of capillary obstruction.

Figure 6 summarises some of these potential causes of capillary obstruction – endothelial cell swelling; plugging by platelet aggregates or activated polymorphonuclear leucocytes; and tissue oedema. As previously noted, $PGI_2$ may play a role in inhibiting such processes: hence infusion of pharmacological doses of prostanoids may overcome "relative $PGI_2$ deficiency" and is one approach to limitation of these interactive processes which favour critical ischaemia. This concept is developed further in Chapter 9.

## 3.5 Conclusion

This chapter has outlined some of the complex disturbances which may occur in critical limb ischaemia, ending with a speculative synthesis of some of these factors. This scheme is meant to provoke discussion and integration of the different approaches of many workers, and it should be appreciated that many of the processes discussed lack direct evidence of their importance in human patients. Acquisition of such evidence is an important future goal in understanding the complex interplay of factors involved in the pathogenesis of critical leg ischaemia.

## References


1. Bird T, Leithead CS, Lowe KG (1954) Symmetrical peripheral gangrene in low output heart failure. Lancet II:780–782
2. Gokal R, Dornan TL, Ledingham JGG (1979) Peripheral skin necrosis complicating beta-blockage. Br Med J I:721–722
3. Mitchell JRA, Schwartz CJ (1965) Arterial disease. Blackwell Scientific, Oxford
4. Fowkes FGR (1988) Epidemiology of atherosclerotic arterial disease in the lower limbs. Eur J Vasc Surg 2:283–291
5. Lowe GDO (ed) (1987) Blood rheology and hyperviscosity syndromes. Baillière's Clin Haematol 1:597–867
6. Strandness DE Jr, Sumner DS (1975) Haemodynamics for surgeons. Grune and Stratton, New York
7. Yao JST (1970) Haemodynamic studies in peripheral arterial disease. Br J Surg 57:761–766
8. Davies MJ, Thomas AC (1985) Plaque fissuring – the cause of acute myocardial infarction, sudden ischaemic death, and crescendo angina. Br Heart J 53:363–373
9. Lowe GDO, Douglas JT, Zahrani H, Pollock JG, Smith WC, Crombie I, Tunstall-Pedoe H (1988) Plasma D-dimer antigen in chronic peripheral arterial disease and in a population study. Fibrinolysis 2 (Suppl) 1:37
10. Carter SA, Lezack JD (1971) Digital systolic pressures in the lower limb in arterial disease. Circulation 43:905–914
11. Gundersen J (1972) Segmental measurements of systolic blood pressure in the extremities including the thumb and the great toe. Acta Chir Scand 426 (Suppl):1–90
12. Fagrell B (1973) Vital capillary microscopy – a clinical method for studying changes of the nutritional skin capillaries in legs with arteriosclerosis obliterans. Scand J Clin Lab Invest 31 (Suppl) 133:1–50
13. Dormandy JA (1989) Personal communication
14. Hirai M, Kawai S (1978) Clinical significance of segmental blood pressure in arterial occlusive disease of the lower extremity. VASA 7:383–388

15. Tønnesen KH (1978) Transcutaneous oxygen tension in imminent foot gangrene. Acta Anaesth Scand 68:107–110
16. Morris-Jones W, Preston E, Greaves M, Duleep K (1981) Gangrene of the toes with palpable peripheral pulses. Ann Surg 193:462–466
17. Fagrell B, Lundberg G (1984) A simplified evaluation of vital capillary microscopy for predicting skin viability in patients with severe arterial insufficiency. Clin Physiol 4:403–411
18. Gundersen J (1972) Segmental measurements of systolic blood pressure in the extremities including the thumb and the great toe. Acta Chir Scand (Suppl):1–90
19. McEwan AJ, Ledingham IM (1971) Blood flow characteristics and tissue nutrition in apparently ischaemic feet. Br Med J III:220–224
20. Bartoli V, Dorigo B, Tedeschi E, Biti GP, Voegelin HR (1970) Circadian periodicity of calf blood flow in subjects with intermittent claudication. Angiology 21:215
21. Conrad MC (1971) Functional anatomy of the circulation to the lower extremities. Year Book Medical Publishers, Inc. Chicago
22. Franzeck UK, Isenring G, Frey J, Bollinger A (1983) Videodensitometric pattern recognition of Na-fluorescein diffusion in nailfold capillary areas of patients with acrocyanosis, primary and secondary Raynaud's phenomenon. Inter Angio 2:143–152
23. Fagrell B (1983) Monitoring the effects of vasoactive drugs by capillaroscopy and capillary blood flow velocity measurement. Int Angio 2:153–158
24. Franzeck UK, Liebethal R, Diehm C (1987) Mikrovaskulare Flußverteilung und transcutaner Sauerstoffpartialdruck der Hautkapillaren von Patienten mit peripherer arterieller Verschlußkrankheit im Stadium III und IV. VASA (Suppl) 20:309–310
25. Franzeck UK, Talke P, Bernstein EF, Golbranson FL, Fronek A (1982) Transcutaneous oxygen tension measurements in health and peripheral arterial occlusive disease. Surgery 91:156–163
26. Karanfilian RG, Lynch TG, Zirul VT, Padberg FT, Jamil Z, Hobson RW (1986) The value of laser Doppler velocimetry and transcutaneous oxygen tension determination in predicting healing of ischemic forefoot ulcerations and amputations in diabetic and nondiabetic patients. J Vasc Surg 4:511–516
27. Hoffman U, Bollinger A (1988) Laser-Doppler. In: Kriesman A (ed) Aktuelle Diagnostik und Therapie in der Angiologie. Thieme, Stuttgart New York, pp 56–60
28. Seifert H, Jager K, Bollinger A (1988) Analysis of flow motion by the Laser Doppler technique in patients with peripheral arterial occlusive disease. Int J Microcirc, Clin Exp 7:223–236
29. Hoffman U, Saesseli B, Geiger M, Schneider E, Bollinger A (1988) Vasomotion in patients with severe ischaemia before and after percutaneous transluminal angioplasty (PTA). Int J Microcirc, Clin Exp, Special Issue, August:89
30. Conrad MC (1968) Abnormalities of the digital vasculature as related to ulceration and gangrene. Circulation 38:568–581
31. Ehrly AM (1976) Therapy of occlusive arterial disease with ancrod. Artery 2:98
32. Reid HL, Dormandy JA, Barnes AJ et al. (1976) Impaired red cell deformability in peripheral vascular disease. Lancet I:666–668
33. Lowe GDO, Reavey MM, Johnston RV, Forbes CD, Prentice CRM (1979a) Increased platelet aggregates in vascular and non-vascular illness: correlation with plasma fibrinogen and effect of ancrod. Thromb Res 14:377–386
34. Nash GB, Thomas PRS, Dormandy JA (1988) Abnormal flow properties of white cells in patients with severe ischaemia of the leg. Br Med J 296:1699–1701
35. Lowe GDO, Prentice CRM (1982) Haemostatic and haemorheological factors in peripheral vascular disease. In: Pollock JG (ed) Topical reviews in vascular surgery, vol 1. Wright, Bristol London Boston, pp 25–48
36. Dormandy JA, Hoare E, Colley J, Arrowsmith DE, Dormandy TL (1973a) Clinical, haemodynamic, rheological and biochemical findings in 126 patients with intermittent claudication. Br Med J IV:576–581
37. Stringer MD, Görög PG, Freeman A, Kakkar VV (1989) Lipid peroxides and atherosclerosis. Br Med J 298:281–284

38. Christe M, Delley A, Marbet GA, Biland L, Duckert F (1984) Fibrinogen, factor VIII related antigen, anti-thrombin III and alpha-2-antiplasmin in peripheral arterial disease. Thromb Haemostas 52:240–242
39. D'Angelo Y, Villa S, Mysllvvlec M, Donati MB, de Gaetano G (1978) Defective fibrinolytic and prostacyclin-like activity in human atheromatous plaques. Thromb Haemostas 39:535–536
40. Lowe GDO, Small M (1988) Stimulation of endogenous fibrinolysis. In: Kluft C (ed) Tissue-type plasminogen activator (t-PA). CRC Press, Boca Raton
41. FitzGerald GA, Smith B, Pedersen AK, Brash AR (1984) Increased prostacyclin biosynthesis in patients with severe atherosclerosis and platelet activation. N Engl J Med 310:1065–1068
42. Mehta J, Lawson D, Metha P, Nichols WW (1987) Leukotriene-induced relaxation of precontracted rat aortic rings: dependence on endothelial integrity. Clin Res 35:573a
43. Gryglewski RJ, Palmer RMJ, Moncada S (1986) Superoxide anion is involved in the breakdown of endothelium-derived vascular relaxing factor. Nature (Lond) 320:454
44. Zahavi J, Zahavi M (1985) Enhanced platelet release reaction, shortened platelet survival time and increased platelet aggregation and plasma thromboxane $B_2$ in chronic obstructive arterial disease. Thromb Haemostas 53:105–109
45. Forconi S, Pieragalli D, Guerrini M, DiPerri T (1987) Hemorheology and peripheral arterial diseases. Clin Hemorheol 7:145–158
46. Hess H, Mietasch KA, Deischel G (1985) Drug-induced inhibition of platelet function delays progression of peripheral occlusive arterial disease. Lancet I:415–419
47. Clagett GP, Genton E, Salzman EW (1989) Antithrombotic therapy in peripheral vascular disease. Chest 95 (Suppl) 128S–139S
48. Lowe GDO, Morrice JJ, Forbes CD et al. (1979b) Subcutaneous ancrod therapy in peripheral arterial disease: improvement in blood viscosity and nutritional blood flow. Angiology 30:594–599
49. Kretschmer G, Wenzl E, Schemper M et al. (1988) Influence of postoperative anticoagulant treatment on patient survival after femoropopliteal vein bypass surgery. Lancet I:797–799
50. Ernst E, Hammerschmidt DE, Bagge U, Matrai A, Dormandy JA (1987) Leukocytes and the risk of ischemic diseases. JAMA 257:2318–2324
51. Ross R (1986) The pathogenesis of atherosclerosis. N Engl J Med 314:488–500
52. Mehta P, Mehta J, Lawson D, Krop I (1986) Leukotrienes potentiate the effects of epinephrine and thrombin on human platelet aggregation. Thromb Res 41:731–738
53. Dinerman J, Mehta J, Lawson D, Mehta P (1988) Enhancement of human neutrophil function by platelets. Thromb Res 49:509–517
54. Ciuffetti G, Mannarino E, Pasqualini L, Mercuri M, Lennie SE, Lowe GDO (1988) The hemorheological role of cellular factors in peripheral vascular disease. VASA 17:168–170
55. Ciuffetti G, Balendra R, Lennie SE, Anderson J, Lowe GDO (1989) Impaired filterability of white cells in acute cerebral infarction. Br Med J 298:930–931
56. Lowe GDO, Saniabadi A, Turner A et al. (1986) Studies on haematocrit in peripheral arterial disease. Klin Wochenschr 64:969–974
57. Dormandy JA, Hoare E, Khattab AH, Arrowsmith DE, Dormandy TL (1973b) Prognostic significance of rheological and biochemical findings in patients with intermittent claudication. Br Med J IV:581–583
58. Bailey MJ, Yates CJP, Johnston CLW et al. (1979) Preoperative haemoglobin as predictor of outcome of diabetic amputation. Lancet II:168–170
59. Gilliland E (1989) Personal communication
60. Berridge J (1989) Personal communication
61. Reiger H, Kohler M, Schoop W et al. (1979) Hemodilution (HD) in patients with ischemic skin ulcers. Klin Wochenschr 57:1153–1161
62. Harland WA, Gilbert JD, Steel G, Brooks CJW (1971) Lipids of human atheroma. Part 5. The occurrence of a new group of polar sterol esters in various stages of human atherosclerosis. Atherosclerosis 13:239–246
63. Tooke JE, Milligan DW (1983) Capillary flow velocity in leukaemia. Br Med J 286:518–519

## *Commentary*

*Alfred Bollinger*

Pathophysiology of critical limb ischaemia is characterized by three essential steps: macrovascular wall damage progressing to stenosis or occlusion, collateral development and phenomena at the microvascular level induced by the proximal changes. Moreover, blood flow diversion (haemometakinesia) is also important.

As has been demonstrated by Ross and coworkers [1] *endothelial cell damage* plays an essential role for initiating the wall changes typical for atherosclerosis. The well known risk factors, homocysteine, toxins or viruses seem to trigger gaps or injuries of the endothelial cell lining. Thrombocytes and monocytes cover the defect or attach to the injured cells and release active substances like the platelet derived growth factor which stimulates immigration of smooth muscle cells from the media into the intima.

These lesions as well as fatty streaks are precursors of plaque formation, progressing in part to haemodynamically relevant stenosis. Complete occlusion of a large artery is mainly due to thrombosis of an already narrowed lumen. Alternatives are haemorrhage into plaques and emboli from the heart or from arterial aneurysms.

When a stenosis induces a pathological pressure gradient into the macrocirculation, *collateral vessels* develop and compensate in part for the decreased transport capacity of the main channel. With complete occlusion of a major artery the limb entirely depends on collateral blood flow. Collateral resistance becomes a main determinant of distal perfusion.

Development of collateral vessels requires time. After subacute occlusion of a main artery the resistance is high and decreases slowly. It may be that the resulting ischaemia is severe enough to cause necrosis before an adequate collateral circulation is established. On the other hand occasional spontaneous recovery from "critical ischaemia" is best explained by enhanced transport capacity of collaterals. A rare alternative is reopening of the artery by endogenous thrombolysis. Multilevel disease is associated with collateral resistance arranged in series. It is most likely to cause critical ischaemia.

The pathophysiological phenomenon of *haemometakinesia* [2] or blood flow diversion [3] is especially important in patients with severe ischaemia. When these patients exercise their limbs or when reactive hyperaemia after arterial occlusion is elicited, blood flow increases in the proximal part of the limb but drops in the distal parts to non measurable values [4]. The distal perfusion pressure temporarily decreases to values below 50 mm Hg. Since minor exercise cannot be avoided even by severely ill patients, this mechanism favours the appearance of trophic lesions.

The microvascular changes develop in the low pressure area distal to arterial occlusions. Four important phenomena have been documented in severe foot ischaemia. Fagrell [5] detected areas of the skin *without blood filled capillaries*. These parts are predilection sites for development of ulceration and/or gangrene.

It is not yet established if some of the invisible capillaries are perfused by plasma alone or not at all.

In skin areas of the foot dorsum containing a normal number of blood filled capillaries *distribution of microvascular flow* is not homogeneous. The time difference between filling of the first and last capillaries by Na-fluorescein injected as a tracer (fluorescence videomicroscopy) is significantly delayed compared to healthy controls [6].

The capillaries in severely ischaemic skin areas exhibit *increased permeability* for corpuscular elements (red blood cells [5]), and for the small solute Na-fluorescein [6]. Transcapillary diffusion of the fluorescent tracer is particularly enhanced in diabetics with critical ischaemia. In this metabolic disorder Na-fluorescein diffuses in increased amounts through the capillary wall and the pericapillary halo border, even in the absence of ischaemia [7].

It has been demonstrated recently [8] that *flux motion with high frequency* (about 20 cycles/min) is significantly more prevalent in patients with severe ischaemia than in controls. After successful reopening of large arteries by peripheral transluminal angioplasty and reversal of rest pain or incipient gangrene, the prevalence of these flux waves decreases (unpublished data). It is not yet known if the waves are the consequence of pathological vasomotion in the precapillary arterioles or correlate with centrally mediated phenomena.

## References

1. Ross R (1986) The pathogenesis of atherosclerosis – an update. N Engl J Med 314:488–500
2. De Bakey ME, Burch GE, Ray T, Ochsner A (1974) The "borrow-lending" haemodynamic principle (hemometakinesia) and its application in peripheral vascular disturbances. Ann Surg 126:850
3. Winsor T, Hyman C, Payne JH (1959) Exercise and limb circulation in health and disease. Arch Surg 78:184
4. Bollinger A, Barras JP, Mahler F (1976) Measurement of foot artery blood pressure by micromanometry in normal subjects and in patients with arterial occlusive disease. Circulation 53:506–512
5. Fagrell B, Lundberg G (1984) A simplified evaluation of vital capillary microscopy for predicting skin viability in patients with severe arterial insufficiency. Clin Physiol 4:403–411
6. Jünger M, Frey-Schnewlin G, Bollinger A (1989) Microvascular flow distribution and transcapillary diffusion at the forefoot in patients with peripheral ischemia. Int J Microcirc, Clin Exp 8:3–24
7. Bollinger A, Frey J, Jäger K, Seglias J, Siegenthaler W (1982) Patterns of diffusion through skin capillaries in patients with long-term diabetes. N Engl J Med 307:1305–1310
8. Seifert H, Jäger K, Bollinger A (1988) Analysis of flow motion by the Laser Doppler technique in patients with peripheral arterial occlusive disease. Int J Microcirc, Clin Exp 7:223–236

# Chapter 4

# Investigation and General Management

Bengt Fagrell



## 4.1 Assessment and Investigations

Patients with critical limb ischaemia (CLI) usually have generalized atherosclerosis with symptoms from other organs such as the heart and the brain. The prognosis for patients with CLI is very poor, and almost 50% of the patients die within five years of the appearance of symptoms [1–6]. Therefore, it is of utmost importance that the whole vascular system is assessed in these patients. A careful medical history and examination should be performed.

### 4.1.1 Medical History and Status

The *medical history* must include information regarding development, duration and severity of cardiac symptoms. Many of the patients with CLI have a bad prognosis within the next few years mainly because of severe cardiovascular disease. Coronary insufficiency is often present and sometimes surgical intervention on the coronary arteries must precede an operation for the ischaemic limb. It is also recommended that the status of the carotid arteries should be checked in order to take steps to prevent cerebral catastrophes. All risk factors (smoking, hypertension, hyperlipidaemia, diabetes etc.) should also be recorded. (For the clinical significance of other cardiac conditions, see 3.2.1.)

*Drug treatment* for all other diseases should be checked, especially betablockers which may have a negative influence on the symptoms in the leg with *critical* ischaemia [7, 8], and may decrease the microcirculation in the ischaemic area.

*Inspection of the leg and the whole foot* is important and one should look for discolouration, ulcers, loss of hair on toes etc. An *elevation test* is recommended, and should be performed by elevating the leg 45° above the horizontal level. The patient should then be asked to perform dorsal and plantar movements of the foot for about one minute. The test is positive if the foot becomes pale after this procedure. To increase the sensitivity of the test the patient should be asked to sit up with the leg in a dependent position. The ischaemic leg will then often become more red than the non-ischaemic one, and after some minutes also warmer. *Palpation of the pulses* in the femoral, popliteal, posterior tibial, and dorsalis pedis arteries should be performed. It should be observed that the dorsalis pedis artery is absent in about 10% of the healthy population! The radial, ulnar and carotid arteries should also be examined. In *diabetic patients* examination must also include a full neurological assessment. This should include pain, temperature, touch, vibration sense and reflexes.

R 3

### 4.1.2 Clinical Physiological and Laboratory Investigations

*Cardiovascular System*

As has already been mentioned, coronary atherosclerosis is very often present in patients with CLI. In a recent Swedish study more than 40% of the patients with CLI had symptoms of angina pectoris [6]. In about 10% of the patients there were also symptoms of atherosclerosis in the carotid and cerebral arteries. About 40% of the patients had treatment for hypertension. A resting ECG should therefore be performed to rule out severe coronary insufficiency or arrhythmia. A chest X-ray should also be taken to look for subclinical cardiac failure, obstructive lung diseases, excessive calcifications or carcinoma. It is of extreme importance to optimise treatment for angina pectoris or cardiac failure in patients with CLI. The primary reason for this is that an improved central circulation will also lead to an improvement of the peripheral circulation of the ischaemic limb. Optimal treatment of the cardiovascular system is also of great importance if the patient is going to have an operation.

*Peripheral Macrocirculation*

As the primary cause of symptoms in patients with CLI is most often stenoses or occlusions of the main leg arteries, a careful mapping of the peripheral arterial system is essential. Several non-invasive techniques are now available for this purpose, and the most often used are *segmental blood pressure measurement* and *oscillography*. By these techniques the severity and location of the arterial obliterations can be evaluated. It should be stressed that severe calcification will sometimes make it difficult, or even impossible, to compress the lower leg arteries, making the ankle pressure in these patients artificially high. This is the case in about 10% of diabetics. In these patients the oscillometric index is more useful.

It should also be stressed that if vascular surgery or interventional radiology (e.g. PTA) is considered, the patient must have an *angiogram* of the abdominal aorta down to the foot in order to determine the possibility of such procedures. If a department of radiology is not available at the hospital the patient should be

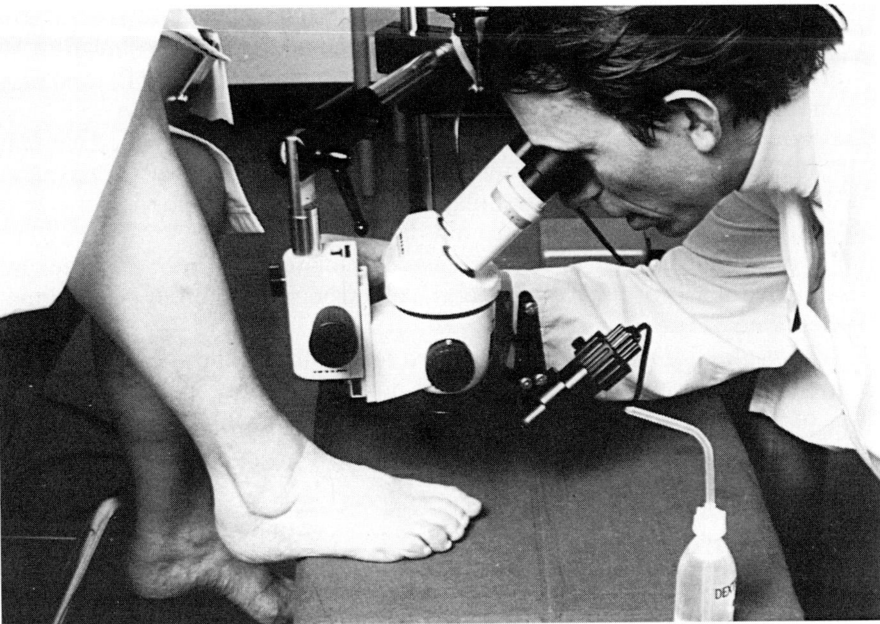

**Fig. 1.** By a simple stereo-microscope with a magnification of 10 to 50 × the morphology of the nutritional skin capillaries can be directly evaluated in ischaemic regions of patients with critical limb ischaemia. The morphological changes of the capillaries can be classified and the risk of skin necrosis developing evaluated (see Section 3.2.3)

referred to a unit for angiography as fast as possible. In patients with CLI a delay of even a day or two may be detrimental and lead to a marked deterioration of the necrotic skin lesions. A mapping of the whole arterial system down to the foot arteries is important, as the state of the distal arteries, i.e. the *run off*, may strongly influence the prognosis after a vascular reconstruction [9].

*Local Skin Microcirculation*

As the final cause for the symptoms in patients with CLI is a marked reduction or abolition of the nutritional circulation in the area, it is necessary to use microcirculatory methods for evaluating the nutritional status of the local skin [10, 11]. During the past few years various new methods have been developed for this purpose.

*Vital capillaroscopy* is a technique with which the blood filling and morphology of the nutritional skin capillaries can be directly and non-invasively evaluated in clinical practice (Fig. 1). As ulcers are most often localized to limited areas, like a toe, it is necessary to use a technique that can map the microcirculation of the whole foot. This can be performed by capillaroscopy. It has been shown that if a normal structure and blood filling of the capillaries are seen in the skin, the risk of necrosis developing is less than 10% during an observation period of three months, regardless of the macrocirculatory status [12]. However, if marked destruction of the capillary bed is present and no blood enters the nutritional capillaries in the sitting position, there is almost a 100% risk of skin necrosis developing over the same period. The technique has been shown to be very valuable for predicting the risk of skin ulcers in patients with CLI, and also for evaluating the prognosis of ischaemic foot ulcers [12] (Section 3.2.3).

*Laser Doppler fluxmetry,* a method which mainly evaluates the blood circulation through the non-nutritional thermoregulatory vascular plexus of the skin, can also be used to give a rough estimation of the microcirculation in the area [13, 14]. However, it should be pointed out that the technique does not seem to be useful for predicting the risk of skin necrosis developing, most probably because it does not give any information whether the blood comes out into the nutritional capillaries or not [15].

*$TcPO_2$ measurements* have also been used for evaluating the reduction of skin circulation [16]. However, this method does not seem to be useful for predicting the risk of skin necrosis, but if it is combined with inhalation of oxygen it has been shown to be a good predictor for determining the appropriate amputation level [17].

*Bood Tests*

The prognosis for the ischaemic leg has been shown to be strongly influenced by different components in the blood [18]. Therefore a full analysis of the blood should be performed including ESR or plasma viscosity, prothrombin time and fibrinogen. It has been shown in several studies that the haemoglobin value, the fibrinogen level, and the number of platelets and leucocytes are very strong predictors for the fate of the ischaemic leg, e.g. after vascular reconstructive surgery [18, 19].

R 4 *Additional Optimal Investigations*

As has been pointed out earlier, it is of great importance to assess the whole cardiovascular system for optimising the central circulation. An exercise ECG may be useful for evaluating the status of the coronary arteries and for deciding whether a coronary angiogram should be performed. However, patients with CLI can seldom perform a bicycle or walking test, but these patients can do an arm exercise test instead.

For the investigations of the peripheral macrocirculation Doppler wave form analysis of the peripheral arteries may be helpful. The new technique of Duplex scanning for looking at the femoral and iliac arteries may also be valuable, and can give detailed information of the flow dynamics of these arteries. In the more distal arteries of the leg the resolution is not very good.

## 4.2 General Management

As has been pointed out earlier a large number of patients with CLI have other coexisting diseases, especially from the cardiovascular and renal systems. Lung diseases, such as chronic bronchitis or bronchial carcinoma also often occur in these patients due to the high proportion of smokers. *It is therefore obligatory to inform the patient strongly of the necessity to stop smoking*. We know from several studies that both the macro- and microcirculation of ischaemic areas may be improved by abolishing smoking [4, 20, 21]. The main reason for this is that the rheological properties of the blood improves with concomitant improvement of the nutritional skin circulation [22]. In normal skin the blood flow is decreased by smoking, but whether this is also the case in ischaemic areas where the microvascular bed is dilated and the reactivity significantly disturbed is not known [23].

### 4.2.1 Coronary Heart Disease

Co-existing coronary insufficiency is present in the majority of patients with CLI. R 5
It is therefore important to evaluate the coronary circulation with, for instance, an exercise test in order to reveal the necessity and possibility of the patient requiring coronary bypass surgery before arterial surgery is performed. R 7
Other severe cardiac symptoms such as heart failure should be optimally treated. Oedema in the ischaemic area is deleterious for the nutritional circulation and must be intensively treated [10].

### 4.2.2 Hypertension

Blood pressure should be controlled to normal levels in patients with severe 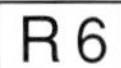

artherosclerosis. However, in the early phase of CLI an elevated blood pressure may be beneficial for the perfusion of the ischaemic region, and blood pressure

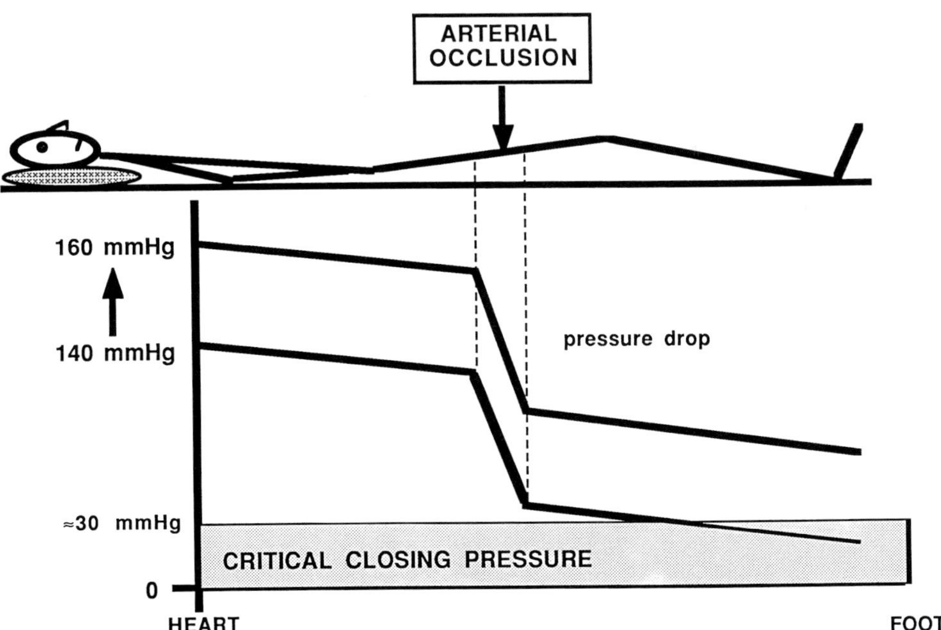


**Fig. 2.** Graphic demonstration of how an increase in the systemic blood pressure of 20 mm Hg (140–160 mm Hg) may have a beneficial effect on the local circulation of an ischaemic area. In the present example the *critical closing pressure* would be overcome, with an improvement of the nutritional circulation of the area

treatment in these patients may be postponed if the blood pressure remains within the limits of *180 over 100 mm Hg* in the sitting or standing position. If the systemic blood pressure is increased by 10 mm Hg, the local blood pressure of the ischaemic region will most probably also be elevated by 10 mm Hg. Such an increase of the local blood pressure may occasionally be enough to markedly improve the nutritional circulation of the ischaemic area (Fig. 2). If antihypertensive drugs must be given, betablockers should be avoided as these drugs have been shown sometimes to have deleterious effects on skin circulation in ischaemic areas [7, 8, 24]. Angiotensin-converting enzyme inhibitors, calcium-antagonists or other vasodilating substances should be used instead.

### 4.2.3 Infection

One of the most serious threats to patients with CLI is bacterial infection. In order to avoid this, the area *should be kept dry*. If the skin around the ulcer can be kept dry, the risk of bacteria infiltrating the surrounding tissue is reduced, while if wet bandages are used the skin is macerated with an increased risk for spreading the infection. Mechanical cleaning of the ulcer area and removal of dead necrotic material is necessary.

R 8 It should be borne in mind that an infection can extend rapidly in an ischaemic area and *antibiotics* should therefore be instituted immediately when signs of infection are present. The antibiotics should be used systemically and be administered intravenously for a speedy effect. In some countries the intra-arterial route is prefered as this is believed to produce higher tissue concentrations.

### 4.2.4 General Management of the Ischaemic Limb

When rest pain and ulcers are present in the foot, the patient should avoid walking on the diseased limb, as this may harm the vulnerable ischaemic tissue. In or-
R 9 der to improve the transmural pressure it is recommended that the ischaemic foot
is kept in the lowest possible position, without inducing oedema. When the foot is in a dependent position, the patient should be instructed to practise calf muscle

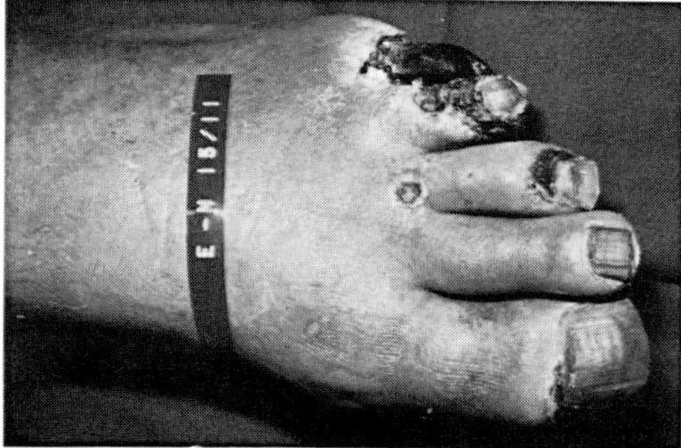

**Fig. 3.** Skin necrosis in patients with PAOD is often initiated by pressure from shoes. The ulcers of this diabetic patient with neuroischaemia was precipitated by trauma from too narrow shoes, and the ulcers are typically located at the edge of the foot in the first, fourth and fifth toes

contractions in order to help the blood return to the heart, minimizing the risk of oedema formation. If oedema is present it has to be treated by diuretics, preferably a loop diuretic, for example furosemide. It has been shown that oedema, especially in diabetics, may totally compress the nutritional skin capillaries in ischaemic areas so that they become completely devoid of blood cells [10, 25]. By reducing the oedema in such areas the blood may enter the capillaries again, with a concomitant improvement, and even healing of an ischaemic ulcer.

*Footcare.* Ulcers or necroses in CLI are most frequently observed in the first, second and fifth toes [25, 26]. Frequent occlusions of the precapillary arterioles (30–50 μm) and empty capillaries have been found in these toes in patients with CLI. This is most probably due to differences in local pressure and trauma, as from shoes (Fig. 3). Even the slightest pressure from a shoe may damage the ischaemic tissue and completely block the blood from entering the nutritional skin capillaries, and consequently induce an ulcer. It is therefore of utmost importance to recommend patients to have shoes large enough not to touch the skin of the acral parts of the feet. Thick, foam rubber inner soles should be used in order to distribute the pressure over the foot more evenly during walking.

## References


1. Silbert S, Zazeela H (1958) Prognosis in arteriosclerotic peripheral vascular disease. JAMA 166:1816–1821
2. Kannel WB, Shurtleff D (1971) The natural history of atherosclerosis obliterans. In: Gifford RW (ed) Peripheral vascular disease. Philadelphia (Cardiovascular clinics; vol III), pp 38–52
3. Stoney RJ (1978) Ultimate salvage for the patient with limb-threatening ischemia. Am J Surg 136:228–232
4. Hughson WG, Mann JI, Tibbs DJ, Woods HF, Walton IB (1978) Intermittent claudicatio: factors determining outcome. Br Med J 1:1377–1379
5. Dormandy J, Thomas P (1988) What is the natural history of a critically ischaemic patient with and without his leg? In: Greenhalgh RM, Jamieson CW, Nicolaides AN (eds) Limb salvage and amputation for vascular disease. WB Saunders Co, London, pp 11–26
6. Bolin T, Aldman Å, Gustavsson P-O, Karlqvist P-Å, Stenberg B, Elfström J (1989) Hur går det för patienter med viloischemi som ej opereras? Läkartidningen 85:2398–2399 (In Swedish only)
7. Gokal R, Dornan TL, Ledingham JGG (1979) Peripheral skin necrosis complicating betablockade. Br Med J 1:721–722
8. Diehm C (1984) Effects of beta-adrenergic blocking drugs on arterial blood flow. VASA 13:201–206
9. Johnston KW, Maureen Rae RN, Hogg-Johnston SA, Colapinto RF, Walker PM, Baird RJ, Sniderman KW, Kalman P (1987) 5-year result of a prospective study of percutaneous transluminal angioplasty. Ann Surg 206:403–413
10. Fagrell B (1977) The skin microcirculation and the pathogenesis of ischemic necrosis and gangrene (Editorial) Scand J Clin Lab Invest 37:473–476
11. Fagrell B (1984) Microcirculation of the skin, chapter VI. In: Mortillaro AN (ed) The physiology and pharmacology of the microcirculation. Academic Press, Baltimore, pp 133–180
12. Fagrell B, Lundberg G (1984) A simplified evaluation of vital capillary microscopy for predicting skin viability in patients with severe arterial insufficiency. Clin Physiol 4:403–411
13. Kvernebo K (1988) Laser Doppler flowmetry in evaluation of lower limb atherosclerosis. Thesis, Aker Hospital, Oslo. Holstad Grafisk A/S, Oslo, Norway

14. Östergren J, Schöps P, Fagrell B (1988) Evaluation of a laser Doppler multiprobe for detecting skin microcirculatory disturbances in patients with obliterative atherosclerosis. Inter Angiol 7:37–41
15. Fagrell B (1989) Peripheral vascular diseases. In: Shepherd AP, Öberg Å (eds) Laser Doppler Flowmetry. Kluwer Academic Publiskers, Norwell, USA (In press)
16. Franzeck U, Talke P, Bernstein EF, Golbrandson FL, Fronek A (1982) Transcutaneous $PO_2$ measurements in health and peripheral arterial occlusive disease. Surgery 91:156–163
17. Harward TRS, Volny J, Golbranson F, Bernstein EF, Fronek A (1985) Oxygen inhalation-induced transcutaneous $PO_2$ changes as a predictor of amputation level. J Vasc Surg 2:220–227
18. Dormandy JA, Hoare E, Colley J, Arrowsmith DE, Dormandy TL (1973) Clinical, haemodynamic, rheological and biological findings in 126 patients with intermittent claudication. Br Med J 4:576–581
19. McCollum CN (1988) Does platelet inhibitory therapy improve vein bypass patency? In: Greenhalgh RM, Jamieson CW, Nicolaides AN (eds) Limb salvage and amputation for vascular disease. WB Saunders Co, London, pp 307–320
20. Department of Health and Human Service (1983) The health consequences of smoking: cardiovascular disease. A report of the surgeon general, Rockville, MD:DHEW, 1–11
21. Cock DG, Pocock SJ, Sharper AG (1986) Giving up smoking and the risk of heart attacks – a report from the British Regional Heart Study. Lancet 2:1376–1380
22. Ernst E, Koenig W, Matrai A, Filipiak B, Stieber J (1988) Blood rheology in healthy cigarette smokers. Results from the MONICA Project, Augsburg, Atherosclerosis 8:385–388
23. Östergren J, Fagrell B (1985) Skin capillary blood cell velocity in patients with arterial obliterative disease and polycythemia – a disturbed reactive hyperemia response. Clin Physiol 5:35–43
24. Greenhalgh RM, Laing SP, Cole PV, Taylor GW (1981) Smoking and arterial reconstruction. Br J Surg 68:605–607
25. Fagrell B (1973) Vital capillary microscopy – a clinical method for studying changes of the nutritional skin capillaries in legs with arteriosclerosis obliterans. Scand J Clin Lab Invest Suppl 133
26. Conrad M (1971) Functional anatomy of the circulation to the lower extremities. Year Book Medical Publishers, Inc. Chicago, USA

## *Commentary*

*Vaughan Ruckley*

It is not easy, in discussing the investigations and management of the vascular patient, to achieve a reasonable balance between a satisfactory minimal standard of care and what would be expected in a major specialist centre or academic unit. Professor Fagrell has outlined an excellent approach from which there can be little dissent.

However it is worth pointing out that one consequence of specialisation (which has been described as knowing more and more about less and less) is that sometimes one loses sight of the whole patient while focussing on the part – in this case the ischaemic part. So perhaps the essence of investigation and management of the patient with critical limb ischaemia (CLI) is retaining a "whole patient" approach and deciding where to draw the line.

For example it would be a pity if the impression were given that something effective can always be done for the patient with CLI. This does not correspond to a considerable proportion of real life situations. This is not an irrelevant digression, since investigations will be limited by projected treatment. As more people survive into the extremes of old age, the vascular surgeon is increasingly consulted on behalf of patients in whom CLI is part of a terminal event, albeit gradual. Often it is best to take no action other than to provide nursing care and whatever analgesia is required to keep the patient comfortable.

Where intractable pain or offensive gangrene are causing distress, amputation without recourse to any specific vascular investigations may be the proper course. The other side of the coin, and probably the more serious one, is the extent to which limbs are being lost unnecessarily without recourse to appropriate investigation, radiological intervention or arterial reconstruction.

Professor Fagrell recommends that the whole vascular system be assessed in patients with CLI. This is entirely reasonable as far as history and examination are concerned. Progress along the investigation pathway is tempered by the appropriateness of "aggressive" interventions in a particular individual. A not uncommon example is the patient whose intractable heart failure means that the cardiac output would be insufficient to sustain a graft, were it attempted. The patient presenting with CLI may already have a flexion contracture at the knee which severely limits the treatment options. Thus, along the investigation pathway that Professor Fagrell has traced, should be a series of decision hurdles demanding careful thought. "Routine" investigations have advantages but do not necessarily lead to appropriate care.

Professor Fagrell rightly emphasises that patients with CLI have a poor prognosis on account of occlusive disease elsewhere, especially in the coronary vessels. At least half of these patients will be dead within five years from myocardial ischaemia. It is clear that the patient with a history of recent myocardial infarction or unstable angina is at considerable risk and none would dispute the need for careful cardiological pre-operative assessment. A distinction needs to be made between investigations aimed at coronary or carotid reconstruction and those employed to assess risk or fitness for operation.

It is rare, in the UK, for patients with CLI to be in an age group in which coronary artery bypass would be seriously considered. The difficulty is to decide how thoroughly to search for coronary disease in the patient with stable, mild or absent cardiac symptoms. Bearing in mind that, by definition, CLI implies that urgent action is essential if a limb is to saved, chest X-Ray, resting ECG and respiratory function tests are all the cardiorespiratory tests that can be said to be routine. Exercise ECG, by treadmill, is impossible in virtually all these patients and many cannot sufficiently raise their cardiac output by means of upper limb activity to make an exercise ECG meaningful. An ejection fraction of less than 30% on radionuclide ventriculogram might contraindicate elective aortic reconstruction, but not necessarily a femoro-popliteal or distal bypass which can be done under regional or even local anaesthesia.

Similar considerations apply to asymptomatic carotid disease. Thus it is an extreme rarity in the UK, in contrast to some centres in North America, to consider coronary or carotid angiography or even Duplex scan as part of the routine assessment of the patient with CLI.

Assessment takes on a different complexion in patients in whom aorto-iliac reconstruction rather than the more usual femoro-popliteal or femoro-distal reconstruction may be required for CLI. Here one is concerned primarily with the patient's ability to survive an abdominal operation and cardiorespiratory function is the main determinant.

Concerning the limb itself, clinical examination is all important and merits some emphasis. To the elevation test described by Professor Fagrell one could add the simple observation of dependent rubor and underline the significance of dependent oedema. Routine measurement of the Doppler ankle pressures is universally helpful provided that the possibilities of observer error are remembered and that undue reliance is not placed on the readings, particularly in diabetics. Segmental pressures and oscillometry are probably only done in those few units in which a vascular technician is regularly available and, like most vascular laboratory tests in critical ischaemia, seldom influence decisions on patient care; these decisions being taken overwhelmingly on the combination of history, physical findings and angiography.

In discussing angiography, Professor Fagrell rightly emphasises the importance of good definition of the run off vessels in the lower calf and foot. This may be difficult to obtain where there are extensive proximal occlusions especially if the cardiac output is impaired. Digital subtraction angiography has a valuable role here, although some surgeons prefer on-table angiography. Non-invasive methods of locating patent distal vessels are also under study [1].

When discussing local care the importance of skilled chiropody should be mentioned. In support of Professor Fagrell's comments on the avoidance of pressure the dangers of anti-embolism stockings and of bandaging should be emphasised [2] especially in diabetics.

Finally Professor Fagrell touches on an important practical area when discussing the position adopted for the critically ischaemic limb. Strong analgesics may be required to subdue rest pain in order to obtain a sufficient elevation, even to near horizontal, for the reduction of oedema and thereby the control of infection. This in turn may increase the ischaemia and, by sedation, depress cardiorespiratory function. It is a vicious circle that can best be averted by early active management of CLI.

### *References*

1. Beard JD, Scott DJA, Evans JM, Skidmore R, Horrocks M (1988) Pulse generated run-off: a new method of determining calf vessels patency. Br J Surg 75:361–363
2. Callam MJ, Ruckley CV, Dale JJ, Harper DR (1987) Hazards of compression treatment of the leg: an estimate from Scottish surgeons. Br Med J 2:295, 138

## Chapter 5

# Percutaneous Reopening Procedures

Wolfgang Krings and Peter E. Peters



## 5.1 Specific Treatment of the Ischaemic Limb

### 5.1.1 Percutaneous Catheter Procedures

Since the introduction of percutaneous transluminal angioplasty (PTA) by Dotter and Judkins [1] in 1964 and the development of the double-lumen balloon catheter by Gruentzig and Hopff [2] in 1974 this method has become established in the treatment of peripheral arterial occlusive disease. It is mainly indicated in isolated stenoses or short occlusions [3] (Fig. 1). The combination of PTA and low-dose local fibrinolysis [4] allows to recanalize even occlusions with unorganized thrombotic material, so that acute and subacute obliterations occurring in the course of chronic arterial occlusion may be treated by means of a catheter (Figs. 2, 3).

The methods can be performed under local anaesthesia and carry a lower risk than surgery [5]. They are, therefore, also appropriate for high-risk patients who can not undergo surgery.

The catheter procedures require a well equipped angiographic suite and a team experienced in angioplasty. Just as with surgical methods and other procedures depending on manual dexterity, the percutaneous catheter procedures can only be successfully performed if sufficient experience has been acquired under guidance (50 to 70 treatments) and if they are regularly carried
out (70 to 100 treatments per year) [3]. For the treatment of peripheral arterial R 17
occlusive disease these methods are used by interventional radiologists, R 18
angiologists and vascular surgeons.

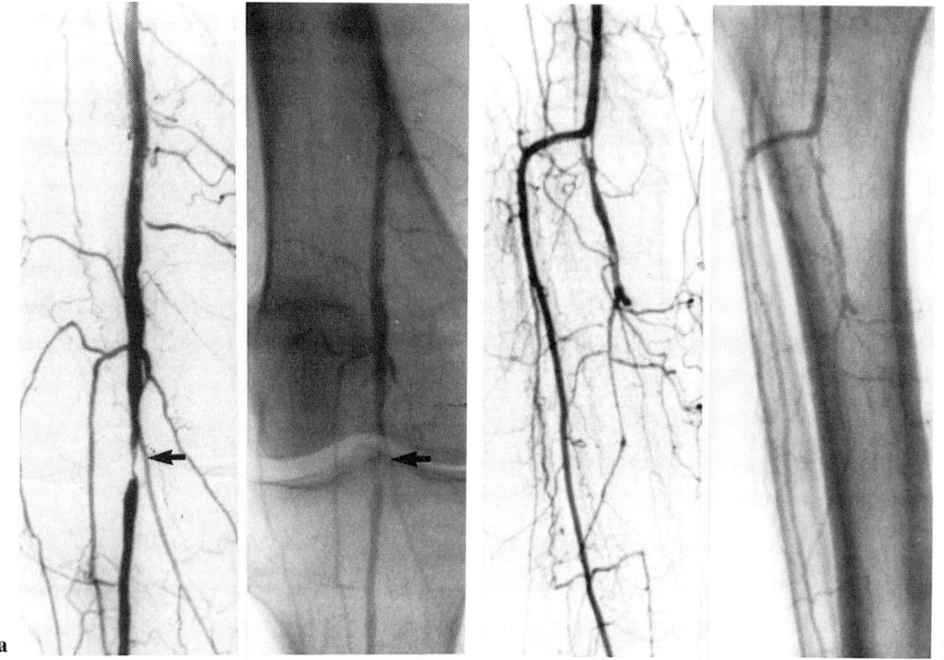

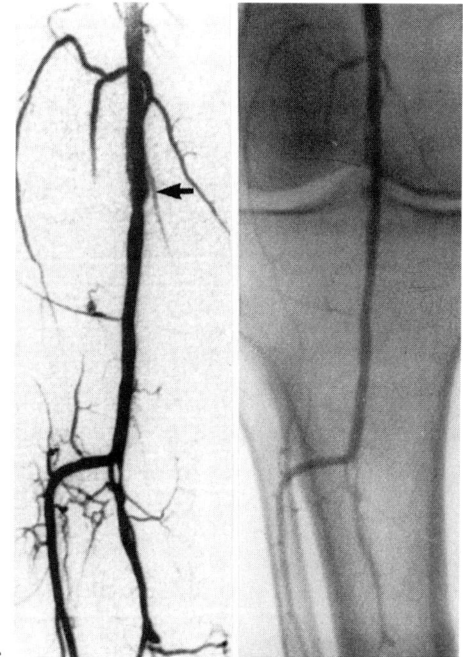

**Fig. 1 a–c.** Chronic peripheral occlusive arterial disease: 59 year old diabetic woman with progressive ischaemic rest pain. **a** Intraarterial DSA of popliteal artery (left); unsubtracted image (right): arteriosclerotic plaques and significant stenosis at the level of the joint cavity (arrow). **b** Intraarterial DSA of proximal leg arteries (left); unsubtracted image (right): stenosis of tibioperoneal trunk, occlusion of peroneal and posterior tibial arteries. **c** Follow-up DSA following successful balloon angioplasty of popliteal artery (left); unsubtracted image (right): angiogram shows only irregular vascular contours without residual stenosis

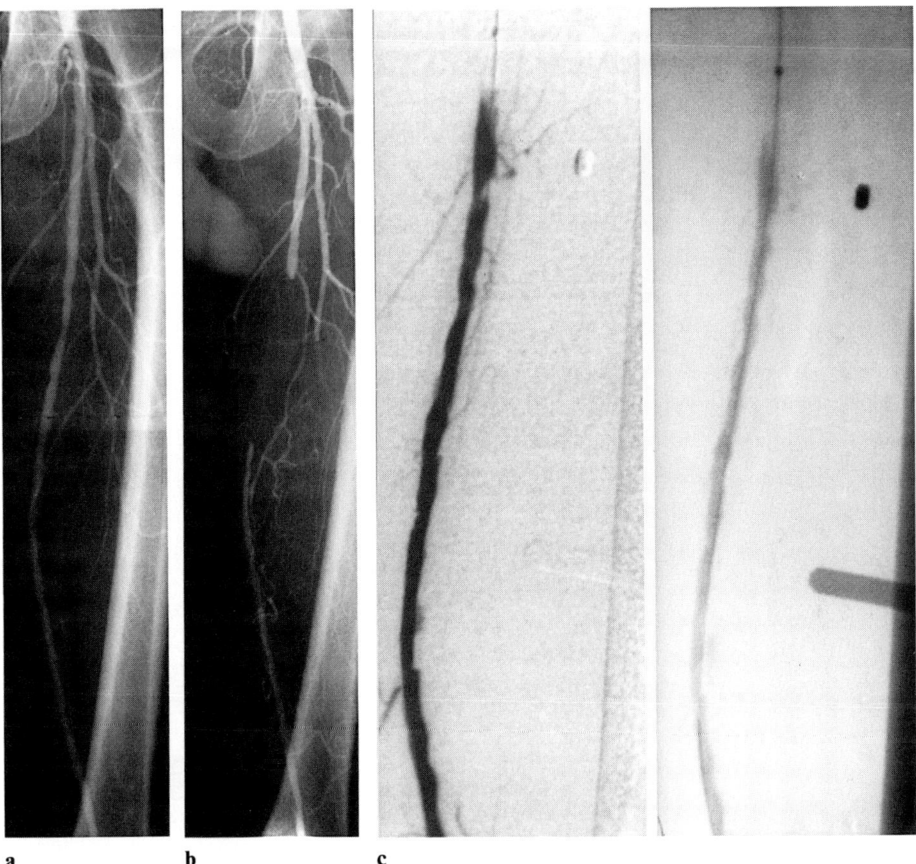


**Fig. 2 a–c.** A 50 year old type I diabetic patient with acute-on-chronic disease and development of toe ulcers: indication for local low-dose fibrinolysis. **a** June 1986: conventional arteriogram shows arteriosclerotic lesions with mild stenoses of superficial femoral artery. **b** December 1989: 14 days after sudden deterioration and development of rest-pain; conventional arteriogram demonstrates an occlusion (9.5 cm of length) in the same region and a poor outflow (stenoses of peroneal and posterior tibial arteries and occlusion of anterior tibial artery). **c** Follow-up DSA after local fibrinolysis with 200000 IU urokinase and balloon angioplasty of preexisting stenoses: patent artery with low grade proximal residual stenosis and irregular vascular contours

### 5.1.1.1 Angioplasty

*Techniques and Indications*

The treatment is performed under local anesthaesia. In most cases, the artery is entered from the ipsilateral femoral artery, puncturing in a retrograde or antegrade direction depending on the localization of the lesion to be treated. In order to reach vascular segments close to the inguinal region or to leave the ipsilateral region undisturbed the cross-over technique is used (Fig. 4). Rarely is it necessary to choose an axillary or popliteal approach. For the treatment of

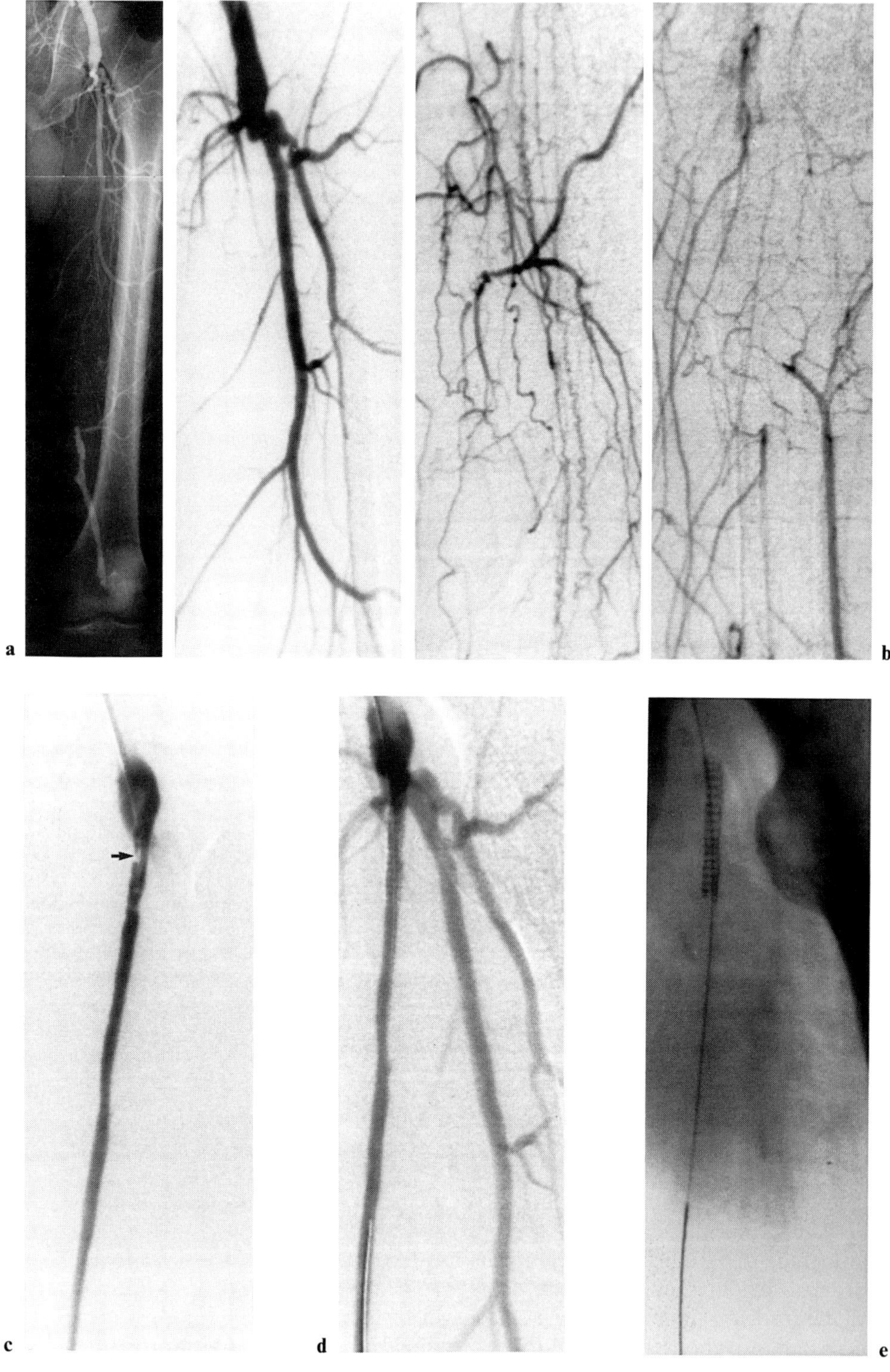
a
b
c
d
e

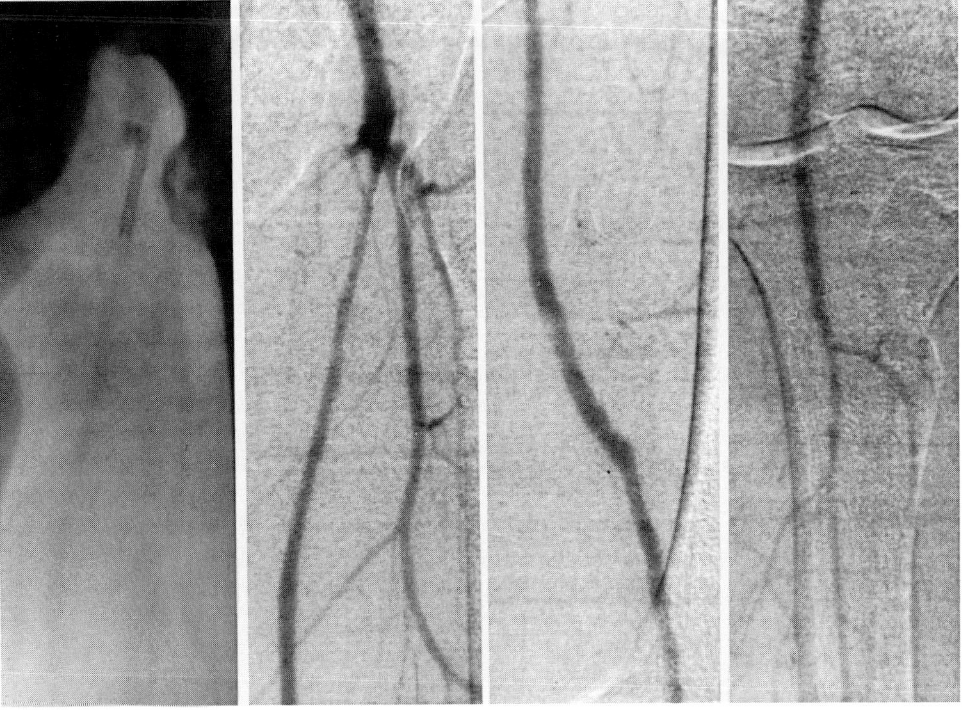

f

**Fig. 3 a–f.** A 53 year old patient with acute-on-chronic disease 3 years following femoropopliteal bypass surgery (venous graft). Mild claudication since 13 months. Acute rest pain developed in November 1989: postoperative catheter treatment in cross-over technique: local low-dose fibrinolysis, balloon angioplasty and stent implantation. **a** conventional angiogram of the left femoropopliteal artery 3 days following the onset of pain: complete occlusion of the bypass and the proximal two thirds of the superficial femoral artery; collateral segmental filling within Hunter's canal; occlusion of the distal popliteal artery. **b** Intraarterial DSA and catheter treatment in cross-over technique 5 days later: total occlussion of the femoropopliteal artery and its trifurcation; collateral filling of the proximal peroneal and anterior tibial arteries. **c** After fibrinolysis of the venous bypass and the femoropopliteal segment with 400 000 IU urokinase, DSA demonstrates the cause of the bypass occlusion: eccentric stenosis just distal of proximal anastomosis; same view after balloon angioplasty showing a valvular type of stenosis. **d** Bridging of stenosis with an intraluminal stent: patent proximal bypass region. **e** Unsubtracted image showing the position of the stent in the left groin. **f** Intravenous DSA 10 days after the intervention: correct stent position, patent bypass, femoropopliteal segment and trifurcation

stenoses of the aorta or the aortal bifurcation the so called kissing-balloon method is recommended.

Generally, the obstruction is first passed with a guide wire and an open-end catheter before the balloon catheter is introduced. Balloon size is determined with reference to a non-stenosed adjacent vascular segment and should not exceed its diameter. Dilatation of the vascular segment to be treated is done under

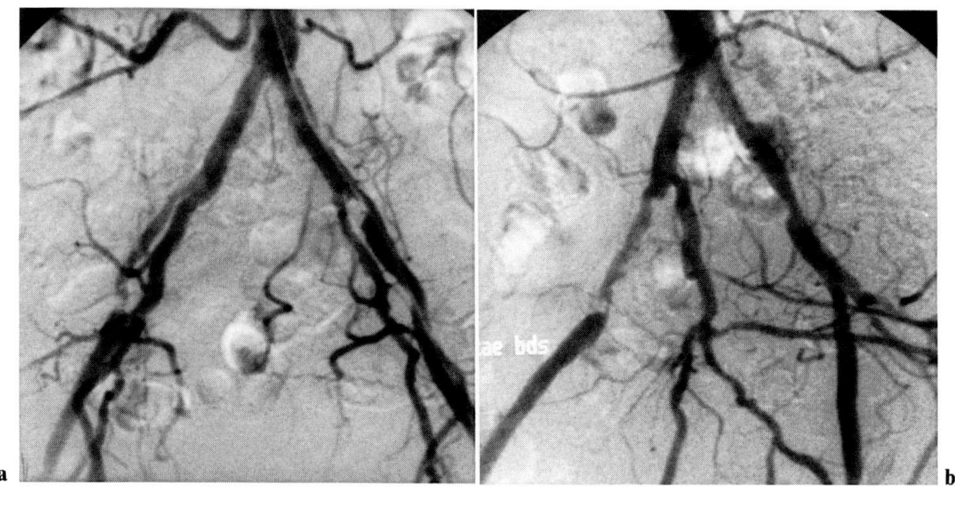


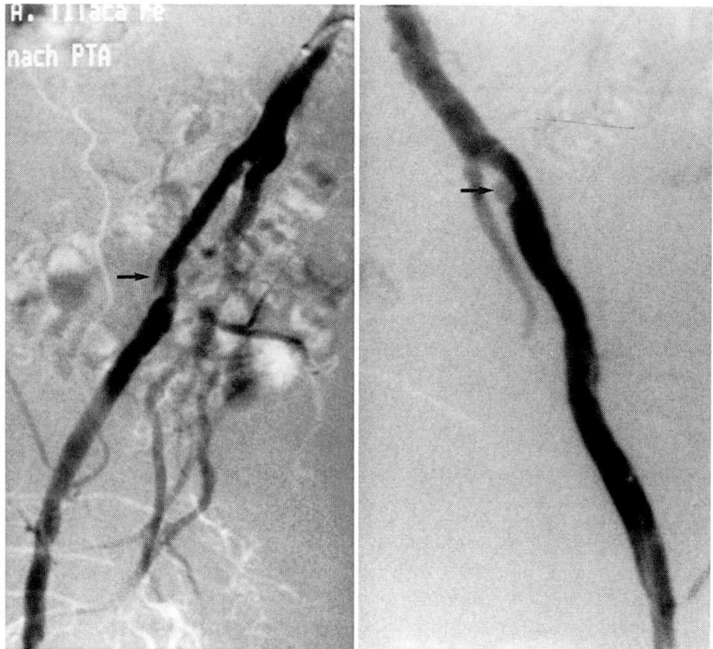


**Fig. 4 a–d.** 74 year old patient with progressive occlusive arterial disease with bilateral external iliac stenosis and long segment femoral occlusion. He had developed a necrotic ulcer on the right big toe within the last three months. For PTA of ipsilateral and contralateral iliac stenoses in the same procedure cross-over technique is recommended. **a** Intraarterial DSA of iliac arteries (AP view): severe stenosis of left external iliac artery at the bifurcation of the common iliac artery; long segment stenosis of right external iliac artery. **b** Oblique view (RPO) demonstrating the extent and the morphology of stenosis. Follow-up angiogram after successful angioplasty: **c** Contralateral (right) iliac artery (PTA in cross-over technique). **d** Ipsilateral (left) iliac artery: arrows indicate wall lesions with bilateral so called intima/media clefts and only mild residual stenosis

fluoroscopic control over a period of 10 to 30 seconds. Balloon catheters currently used have a shaft size of F5 to F8 with a balloon diameter of 4 to 8 mm and balloon length of 20 to 100 mm. Teflon coated, sometimes steerable guide wires are employed. Apart from standard equipment a variety of special wires and catheters is commercially available for the treatment of vessels measuring from 2 to 10 mm in diameter [5, 6].

Aside from conventional angioplasty a growing number of new treatment techniques has been introduced, the value of which has not been clarified so far; their field of application and chance of success cannot be sufficiently judged at the present time. Among these procedures are laser angioplasty, laser or high frequency induced thermal angioplasty, dynamic angioplasty, percutaneous atherectomy and embolectomy, as well as the percutaneous implantation of endovascular prostheses (stents) (Fig. 3). A detailed discussion of these methods will not be given here.

The treatment principle of angioplasty by use of a balloon catheter is based on plaque fracture with or without localized dissection of intima/media [27]. The muscular fibrils of the media are extended and irreparably damaged, leaving permanent local ectasia at the dilation site. Angiography will show a dilated lumen with contrast medium filled clefts within the wall. Over the subsequent weeks and months the resulting necrotic debris is removed by macrophages which results in smoothing of the vascular wall [5].

In view of its mode of action, PTA is particularly appropriate in short obliterations. The main indications today include unilateral or bilateral iliac stenoses (Fig. 4), stenoses of the inguinal artery, isolated or multiple stenoses of the femoral and popliteal artery (Fig. 1), as well as short segment occlusions (<10 cm) of femoropopliteal vessels (Fig. 5). With longer obliterations or infrapopliteal changes a balloon catheter may only be used in strict clinical indications (stage III/IV) and if vascular surgery is contraindicated or less probable to be successful. An additional field of application is the perioperative angioplasty for vascular reconstructions: dilation of iliac stenoses prior to femoropopliteal bypass surgery, improvement of run off, treatment of stenoses in regions of anastomoses (Fig. 3).

Review of the literature shows the highest frequency of PTA indications (65 to 85%) in clinical stage II claudication. The most important clinical indication, however, is decompensated chronic arterial occlusion associated with threatened limb in clinical stages III and IV.

*Disadvantages*

Complication rates of PTA reported in the literature vary considerably. In 1988, Roth et al. [6] reported 3.3% of complications which could be controlled by conservative measures and 0.3% requiring surgery in a total of 2668 angioplasties of pelvic and femoral arteries in his own patient group. Respective values quoted in the literature are 0.76–3.3% complications controlled conservatively and 2.0–3.0% requiring surgery. A mortality rate of 0.2% is given [6].

Considering the group of patients with critical limb ischaemia, a clearly higher rate of complications has to be expected due to compromised general condition, advanced arteriosclerosis, higher age average and frequent accompanying

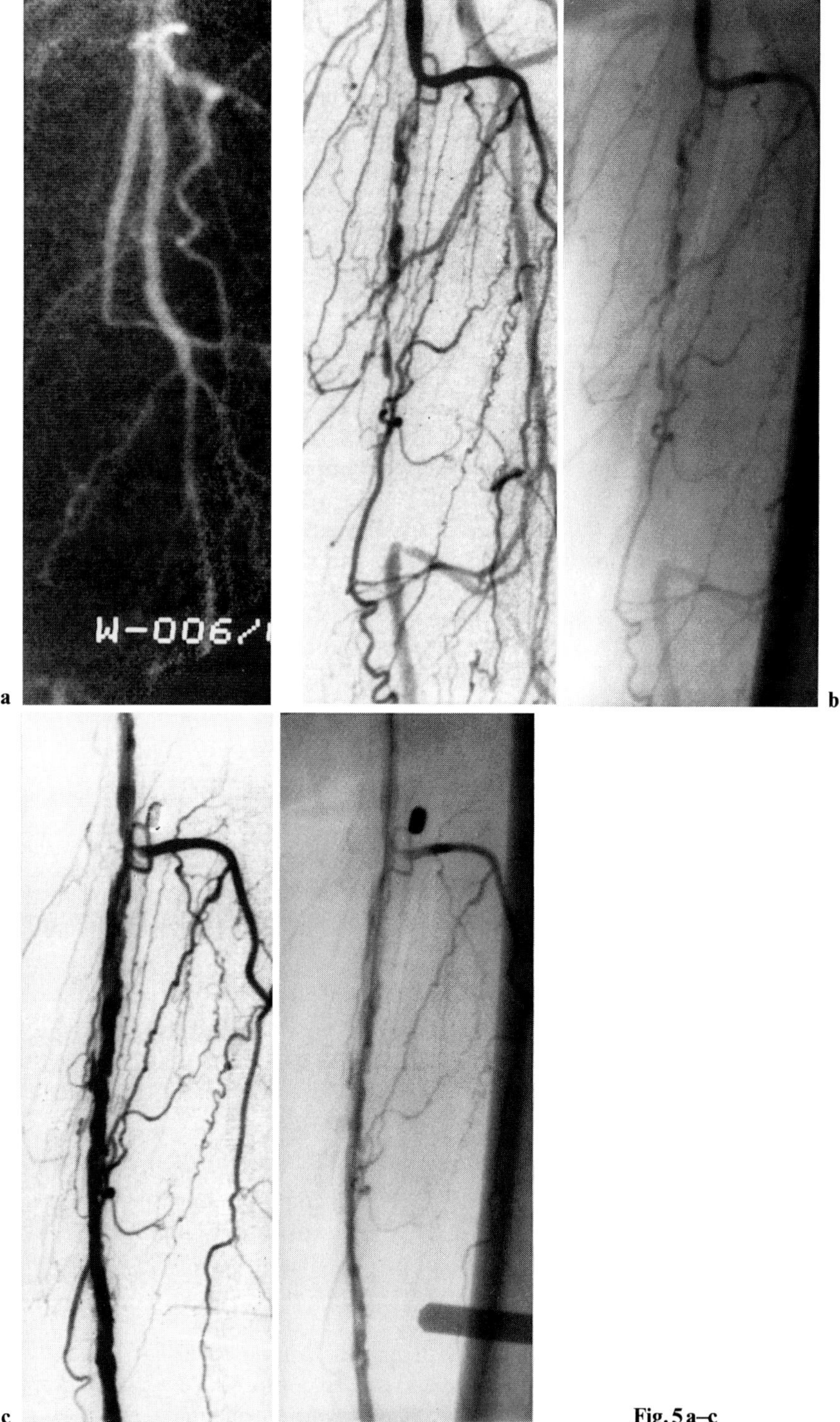


Fig. 5 a–c

diseases. According to Zeitler et al. [7] the rate of surgically treated complications is 1.2% in angioplasties of clinical stage II, but 2.3% in stage III/IV, and is lower in the treatment of pelvic arteries (1.9%) than in the angioplasty of femoropopliteal stenoses (2.7%), short occlusions (2.3%) or occlusions exceeding 10 cm (6.7%). A review of the Anglo-American literature shows complication rates of 3 to 15% in this risk group, and complications requiring surgical intervention of 1 to 5%, a mortality rate of up to 7% is cited. It should be taken into account that these are fairly small groups which cannot be compared directly. Bleeding and thromboembolic events are most often seen. The latter may be lysed locally or aspirated during the same sitting, depending on the severity. Small emboli usually remain asymptomatic and will not be detected even in control angiography some weeks later.

*Contraindications*

The only contraindications to percutaneous transluminal angioplasty given in the literature are uncontrollable coagulation disorders and thrombosis of peripheral aneurysms. Occlusions of pelvic arteries represent a relative contraindication, as the probability of initial success offered by PTA is low (40%) in comparison with surgical vascular reconstruction. Only Cumberland [8] reports an initial success rate of 70%.

Limiting factors are severe obesity, arteries with considerable elongation and sharply kinked arteries, as well as severe calcifications. Antegrade puncture may be impossible in obesity. Sharply kinked arteries usually can be passed and treated with up-to-date catheter material. In the case of occlusions there is a risk of dissection or perforation of the vascular wall. Occlusion situated at the origin of an artery often cannot be probed or passed by guide wire or catheter. Eccentric plaques are frequently resistant to therapy. In these instances percutaneous atherectomy offers new possibilities. Severe calcifications of the vascular wall affects balloon dilatation. There is a higher frequency of media dissections, and the risk of rupture is increased [5].

*Results*

Among the numerous publications on percutaneous transluminal angioplasty published over the last 20 years, there are only few studies on the probability of success with this method in patients with critical limb ischaemia. Above all, there are only few prospective studies with sufficient numbers of patients. The comparison of initial and long-term data is further compromised by differences in statistical evaluation and by different definitions of critical limb ischaemia. No

◄

**Fig. 5 a–c.** 62 year old diabetic female with preexisting chronic arterial occlusive disease of lower leg and rapid clinical deterioration (stage III). **a** Intravenous DSA of left femoral artery: occlusion of superficial femoral artery (10 cm) proximal to the channel of Hunter. **b** Intraarterial DSA after unsuccessful conservative therapy over a period of 3 months (right: unsubtracted image): partially recanalized occlusion with delayed contrast filling of irregular lumen. **c** Control angiography after passage with steerable guide and dilation with balloon catheter (5 mm balloon-diameter): mild proximal residual stenosis, extended wall irregularities after PTA. Good clinical result with mild claudication

publication presents a definition of critical ischaemia consistent with the recommendations of the European Consensus Meeting.

Schmidtke et al. [9] presented one of the first reports on long-term results of percutaneous transluminal angioplasty in clinical stage III/IV, performed in 101 patients with critical limb ischaemia. 71% of their patients treated for stage III, and 40% of those treated for stage IV, could be returned to a stable stage II disease, while amputation had to be performed in 5% (stage III) and 40% (stage IV) over a follow-up period of 6 to 30 months. The treated artery remained patent in only 25.3% of the patients group. The authors conclude that in critical limb ischaemia temporary improvement of circulation will often be sufficient to heal necroses or allow limb-saving marginal amputation.

Schneider et al. [10, 11] report initial success in 79% of a group of 173 stage III and IV patients, and a limb salvage rate after 6 months of 77% in 112 patients followed up. 51% of his patients were diabetics. In all those instances where vascular reopening procedures were unsuccessful amputation of the lower leg or femoral amputation had to be carried out.

Spence et al. [12] published first prospective studies with a cumulative limb salvage rate of 76% after 2 years. Chien-Tai et al. [13] reported initial success in 85% and restenoses within 12 months in 34% of patients, requiring a second angioplasty in 19 cases. After an average follow up period of 13 months, amputation had been prevented in 73%. Similar results have been reported by Lu et al. [14], Rush et al. [15], and Fletcher et al. [16].

Most authors report 10–20% poorer results in critical limb ischaemia than in stage II disease [17, 18]. The same is true for long-term results, which have been published in a prospective study by Johnston et al. [18]; they are 58% in stage III/IV after 6 months, 48% after 1 year, 43% after 2 years, and 33% after 5 years, compared with the stage II results of 85%, 74%, 64%, and 52% for the same time periods. Jones et al. [19] emphasized the comparatively less favorable course in diabetics. With an initial success rate of 81% the treated vessels will still be patent in about 75% of non-diabetics after a period of two years, as opposed to less than 50% in diabetic patients.

In a prospective study Zeitler [3, 20] analyzed 678 stage III/IV patients and 1093 stage II patients treated and followed up for 5 years. 5-year results comparable to those after vascular surgery, have been presented for stenoses of pelvic and femoropopliteal arteries and for short (< 12 cm) obliterations of the superficial femoral and the popliteal artery. Only long femoropopliteal occlusions revealed markedly poorer results. Depending on the sites of obliterations, patients with critical limb ischaemia had 10 to 20% lower patency rates than
R 15 these treated in stage II disease.

Glover et al. [21] obtained a limb salvage rate of 71% in cases treated surgically combined with PTA, while PTA as the only measure resulted in a 34% limb salvage rate. Thus, the authors recommend PTA as an adjunct therapy in critical limb ischaemia.

Schwarten and Cutliff [22] treated only infrapopliteal arteries with low-profile catheters and steerable guide wires in 114 chronic ischaemic limbs. In all cases treatment was indicated for threatened limb loss. At 97%, the initial success rate was remarkably high; the cumulative limb salvage rate after 2 years was still 86%.

### 5.1.1.2 Local Thrombolysis by Direct Infiltration with or without Percutaneous Transluminal Angioplasty

Direct application of the fibrinolytic agent (streptokinase or urokinase) into the occluding material allows thrombolysis without the risk of systemic fibrinolysis. It is widely accepted that in chronic arterial occlusive disease lysable components of the thrombus are still found 1 to 12 months after thrombus formation (lower leg arteries 1 month, femoropopliteal arteries up to 6 months, pelvic arteries up to 12 months).

Contraindications are essentially the same as in angioplasty, with recent cerebral infarction and haemorrhage as well as bleeding gastrointestinal ulcers to be added. Due to the negligible systemic effect local lysis can be performed as early as 2 to 3 days after surgery. The procedure is especially appropriate in acute-on-chronic occlusions within the time periods mentioned above, namely occlusions with a high rate of embolism and reobliteration after angioplasty. Fibrinolysis facilitates probing of the occlusion and reduces the risk of penetrating the catheter into the vascular wall. The lysable parts of the occluding material are largely removed, so that balloon dilatation is either no longer necessary or can be restricted to a shorter vascular segment (Fig. 2). The fibrinolytic agent introduced into the thrombus continues to be active for 24 hours, dissolving remnants of the thrombus. The resulting hyperaemia lasting usually more than 24 hours will prevent acute reobliterations. Furthermore, the thromboembolic complications of angioplasty and thrombotic bypass graft occlusions (Fig. 3) may R 16
also be treated by local fibrinolysis [6, 23].

The technique of low-dose fibrinolysis has not been standardized. Treatment is performed under local anaesthesia. The occlusion should be approached proximally to distally. Hess et al. [4] infiltrate the occluding material by softening the proximal end of the occlusion by use of a fibrinolytic agent and subsequently introducing the catheter into the occlusion. They apply repeated single doses of streptokinase (500 to 1000 IU) and pass the catheter stepwise. PTA is added only in cases of persisting haemodynamically active stenoses (Fig. 2). Other authors prefer urokinase for its better tolerance. At the present time there is also the recombinant tissue-type plasminogen activator (rt-PA) available for intra-arterial administration. Multicentre studies are currently investigating to what extent this substance allows better and lower-risk local fibrinolysis [24].

The question has not been clarified whether repeated single doses or continuous infusion of the fibrinolytic agent produce better results. But there is general agreement that lower doses are needed and less systemic activity occurs with direct infiltration of the thrombus than with the catheter left proximal to the occlusion for continuous injection of the fibrinolytic agent. The dose may be reduced even further when thrombotic material is aspirated [25]. Other treatment concepts provide for a 24 to 48 hour arterial fibrinolysis with continuous application for the removal of remaining thrombi.

Hess et al. [23] have recently recommended not to exceed the total dose of 30000 IU to 50000 IU of streptokinase or 100000 IU to 200000 IU of urokinase, as higher dosage may be accompanied by systemic effects.

One disadvantage is the relatively long duration (2–4 h) of local fibrinolysis, especially of longer occlusions. This has an unfavourable effect on patients who are usually in poor general condition and suffer from persistent rest pain. Moreover, the rate of complications as opposed to conventional PTA is increased. Bleeding at the puncture site requiring treatment is reported in 1.5 to 5.3%, clinically significant macroembolism in 7 to 10% and a mortality rate (from retroperitoneal or intracerebral haematomas) of 1.5% is given [6]. These numbers apply to a non-selected group of patients, and as with routine angioplasty might be expected to be much higher in patients with critical limb ischaemia. But detailed discussions of this subject have not been published so far.

The results of local fibrinolysis published in the literature vary considerably due to the inhomogeneous and hardly comparable patient groups. Roth et al. [6] have reported 71% of stage III/IV local lyses in a total number of 304 treatments. The patency rate in this group was 65%, compared with 74% in stage II. Hess et al. [23] have reported initial success in 53.8%, and a cumulative patency rate after 5 years of 58.8%, in 472 thrombotic, up to 6 months old occlusions. The hospital mortality and amputation rate were 1.6 and 1.95%, respectively. In stage III the patency rate after 5 years was 62.5%, and in stage IV only 50.7%, as opposed to 94.7% in stage IIa and 70.2% in stage IIb. Of note were the poorer long-term results in those cases where balloon dilatation was necessary and the occlusion was longer than 25 cm.

Stein et al. [26] have reported on a group of 50 patients with critical limb ischaemia, where vascular surgery could not be performed either for systemic or local reasons. They found that local thrombolysis led to initial success in only 58% of patients and amputation could be prevented in only 34%. The main reasons given for this unfavourable result are absent or insufficient outflow and proximal AV shunts. If these findings are apparent in the pretherapeutic angiogram the authors recommend not to perform local fibrinolysis as a last resort.

### 5.1.1.3 Pharmacological Prophylaxis after Successful Catheter Reopening Procedures

*PTA*

There is general agreement that thromboembolic prophylaxis requires the application of platelet aggregation inhibitors as early as 1 to 3 days before treatment. Most authors recommend continued treatment for at least 6 months especially in the PTA of the femoropopliteal vascular segment. Dosage is controversial, however, since high acetyl salicylic acid (ASA) concentrations inhibit not only the thromboxane but also the prostacyclin ($PGI_2$) synthesis in the endothelial cells. So far, clinical studies reliably proving the efficacy of a low dosage regimen (100 mg ASA/d) have not yet been presented, so that currently a dosage of 500 to 1000 ASA/d is to be recommended. Often, a combination with dipyridamole (100 to 150 mg/d) is applied. Schneider et al. [10] proposing oral anticoagulation present very impressive long-term results. Other authors recommend anticoagulation only in those instances where long occlusions were treated by angioplasty or in severe PTA induced lesions of the vascular wall. The efficacy of a drug treatment for thromboembolic prophylaxis using platelet aggregation inhibitors after PTA of pelvic arteries has not been confirmed by randomized studies. However most authors recommend inhibition of platelet aggregation by ASA. R 19

Depending on the extent of vascular wall lesions, Chien-Tai et al. [13] and others recommend anticoagulation by heparin for the first days following angioplasty to prevent acute thrombotic complications in the initial ("remodelling") phase. They continue follow-up treatment with aggregation inhibitors.

All authors use heparin at a dosage of 5000 U during angioplasty, mostly applying the drug immediately before passing the occlusion. An overview of other pharmacological adjuncts has been compiled by Becker et al. in 1989 [5]. Medication for the prophylaxis of spasms is needed especially in the popliteal artery and the infrapopliteal vessels; nifedipine and nitroglycerin are available for this purpose [22]. Nifedipine should be applied sublingually at a dosage of 10 mg about 10 minutes prior to passage of the occlusion. Nitroglycerin which is intra-arterially applied as bolus at single doses of 100 μg is considered to be a potent spasmolytic agent. Other substances recommended for the treatment of spasms include lidocaine, tolazoline, and laevadosine [6, 20].

*Local Thrombolysis*

Hess et al. [4] recommend pretreatment with inhibitors of platelet aggregation prior to local fibrinolysis and warn against combination with dipyridamole, as combination of this drug with the resulting fibrin split products may lead to severe vasodilation and a fall in blood pressure. During therapy heparin is injected via the catheter if there is the risk of early reobliteration (compromised outflow, lesions of the vascular wall). For follow-up treatment Hess et al. [23] recommend only ASA (330 to 500 mg), sometimes combined with dipyridamole (75 mg). Other authors apply heparin at therapeutic doses and introduce overlapping oral anticoagulation. Clinical studies supporting superiority of one or the other method have not been presented so far.

#### 5.1.1.4 Future Developments

Recent developments in percutaneous transluminal angioplasty have shown promising early results particularly for the recanalisation of extensive vascular occlusions. Mechanical techniques such as the dynamic Kensey-catheter [28], the Kaltenbach-Vallbracht-rotating catheter [29] and the pulsating guide wire are capable of seeking the path of least resistance through an occlusion, thus establishing a lumen allowing further balloon angioplasty. High energy-angioplasty techniques (laser assisted balloon angioplasty, direct laser angioplasty, radiofrequency angioplasty) have shown encouraging results in both short and long segmental occlusions [30–32]. An interesting new aspect offered by percutaneous atherectomy [36] is the histological analysis of atheromatous material obtained, which may indicate the possible pathomechanism of reocclusion [33].

Early results achieved with percutaneously introducable extendable intraluminal prostheses (stents) are already evident, however the long term results have yet to be investigated [34, 35].

No reliable evidence exists regarding the efficiency of all the new angioplasty techniques described. The need for controlled, randomized, multicentre studies in order to establish criteria for therapeutic protocols is obvious.

## 5.2 Conclusion

PTA is an established effective low-risk alternative to vascular surgery for the treatment of appropriate arterial lesions in patients with arterial occlusive diseases and critical limb ischaemia. Ideal for catheter treatment are single or multiple short stenoses, but also occlusions up to 10 cm. PTA also can be used in combination with reconstructive surgery. It is sometimes performed as a final alternative to amputation in patients totally unfit or unsuitable for reconstructive
R 15 surgery.

Local fibrinolysis extends the spectrum of indications of catheter treatment to acute-on-chronic obliterations, long segment occlusions, occlusions of popliteal trifurcation, complications of PTA and thrombotic reobliterations after
R 16 angioplasty and bypass surgery.

The primary results in critical limb ischaemia reported in the literature are about 10 to 20% poorer than in stage II disease. A limb salvage rate within the first 6 months of 70 to 85% is quoted.

It is apparent in the literature that comparable results are not available, confirming the need of planning and conducting multicentre studies in order to define indications and determine results under standardized conditions in the treatment of as homogeneous a patient group as possible.

## References


1. Dotter CT, Judkins MP (1964) Transluminal treatment of arteriosclerotic obstruction. Description of a new technique and a preliminary report of its application. Circulation 30:654
2. Grüntzig A, Hopff H (1974) Perkutane Rekanalisation chronischer arterieller Verschlüsse mit einem neuen Dilatationskatheter. Modifikation der Dotter-Technik. Dtsch Med Wochenschr 99:2502
3. Zeitler E (1985) Primary and late results of percutaneous transluminal angioplasty (PTA) in iliac and femoro-popliteal obliterations. Inter Angio 4:81
4. Hess H, Mietaschk A, Ingrisch H (1980) Niedrig dosierte thrombolytische Therapie zur Wiederherstellung der Strombahn bei arteriellen Verschlüssen. Dtsch Med Wochenschr 105:787
5. Becker GJ, Katzen BT, Dake MD (1989) Noncoronary angioplasty. Radiology 170:921
6. Roth F-J, Heimig T, Berliner P, Grün B, Koppers B, Krings W (1988) Perkutane Gefäßrekanalisation peripherer Gefäße. In: Günther RW, Thelen M (eds) Interventionelle Radiologie. Thieme, Stuttgart New York, p 20
7. Zeitler E, Richter EI, Roth F-J, Schoop W (1982) Results of percutaneous transluminal angioplasty. Radiology 146:57
8. Cumberland DC (1982) Percutaneous angioplasty in complete iliac occlusions. VASA 11:297
9. Schmidtke I, Roth F-J, Schoop W, Cappius G (1980) Perkutane transluminale Katheterbehandlung bei Kranken mit arteriellen Durchblutungsstörungen im Stadium III und IV. In: Müller-Wiefel H (ed) Mikrozirkulation und Blutrheologie – Therapie der arteriellen Verschlußkrankheit. Verlag Gerhard Witzstrock, Baden-Baden Köln New York, p 411

10. Schneider E, Grüntzig A, Bollinger A (1982) Die perkutane transluminale Angioplastie (PTA) in den Stadien III und IV der peripheren arteriellen Verschlußkrankheit. VASA 11:336
11. Schneider E, Grüntzig A, Bollinger A (1983) Percutaneous transluminal angioplasty for limb salvage – progress in therapy for severe leg ischemia with rest pain and gangrene. In: Dotter CT, Grüntzig A, Schoop W, Zeitler E (eds) Percutaneous transluminal angioplasty. Springer, Berlin Heidelberg New York, p 222
12. Spence RK, Freiman DB, Gatenby R, Hobbs CL, Barker CF, Berkowitz HD, Roberts B, McLean G, Oleaga J, Ring EJ (1981) Long-term results of transluminal angioplasty of the iliac and femoral arteries. Arch Surg 116:1377
13. Chien-Tai L, Zarins CK (1983) Limb salvage by percutaneous transluminal angioplasty. In: Castaneda-Zuniga W (ed) Transluminal angioplasty. Thieme-Stratton Inc, New York, p 127
14. Lu C-T, Zarins CK, Yang C-F, Turcotte JK (1982) Percutaneous transluminal angioplasty for limb salvage. Radiology 142:337
15. Rush DS, Gewertz BL, Lu CT, Ball DG, Zarins CK (1983) Limb salvage in poor-risk patients using transluminal angioplasty. Arch Surg 118:1209
16. Fletcher JP, Fermanis GG, Little JM, Kershaw LZ (1988) The role of percutaneous transluminal angioplasty and femoropopliteal bypass in patients with threatened limb. J Vasc Surg 8:226
17. Creutzig A, Luska G, Elgeti H, Alexander K (1983) Perkutane transluminale Angioplastie der unteren Extremitäten im fortgeschrittenen Lebensalter. Dtsch Med Wochenschr 108:1543
18. Johnston KW, Raew M, Hogg-Johnston SA, Colapinto RF, Walker PM, Baird RJ, Sniderman KW, Kalman P (1987) 5-year result of a prospective study of percutaneous transluminal angioplasty. Ann Surg 206:403
19. Jones BA, Maggisano R, Robb C, Saibil EA, Witchell SJ, Harrison AW (1985) Transluminal angioplasty: results in high-risk patients with advanced peripheral vascular disease. Can J Surg 28:150
20. Zeitler E (1986) Transluminal catheter dilatation. Indications, technical aspects, results. Inter Angio 5:137
21. Glover JL, Bednick PJ, Dilley RS, Becker GB, Richmond BC, Yune HY, Holden RW (1983) Balloon catheter dilatation for limb salvage. Arch Surg 118:557
22. Schwarten DE, Cutliff WB (1988) Arterial occlusive disease below the knee: treatment with percutaneous transluminal angioplasty performed with low-profile catheters and steerable guide wires. Radiology 169:71
23. Hess H, Mietaschk A, Brucki R (1987) Peripheral arterial occlusions: a 6-year experience with local low-dose thrombolytic therapy. Radiology 163:753
24. Verstraete M, Hess H, Mahler F, Mietaschk A, Roth F-J, Schneider E, Baert AL, Verhaeghe R (1988) Femoro-popliteal artery thrombolysis with intraarterial infusion of recombinant tissue-type plasminogen activator – report of a pilot trial. Eur J Vasc Surg 2:155
25. Starck E, McDermott J, Crummy A, Turnipseed W, Achter C, Burgess J (1985) Percutaneous aspiration thromboembolectomy. Intervent Radiol 156:61
26. Stein U, Amendt K, Wagner E, Hild R (1987) Catheter lysis in advanced peripheral OAD – procedure of choice or last resort? VASA 16:358
27. Block PC (1985) The mechanism of transluminal angioplasty. Inter Angio 4:77
28. Kensey RK, Nash JE, Abrahams C, Zarins ChK (1987) Recanalization of obstructed arteries with a flexible, rotating tip catheter. Radiology 165:387–389
29. Vallbracht C, Liermann D, Prignitz I, Süss B, Awiszus H, Paasch C, Landgraf H, Beinborn W, Stickelmann G, Kollath J, Roth F-J, Schoop W, Breddin HK, Kaltenbach M (1989) Rotationsangioplastik – Wiedereröffnung chronischer Arterienverschlüsse mit einem langsam rotierenden Katheter. Klinische Ergebnisse bei 100 Patienten. Fortschr Röntgenstr 151:523
30. Sanborn TA (1989) Technical success, clinical success, and patency in laser angioplasty. Radiology 170:576
31. Heintzen MP, Neubaur T, Klepzig M, Strauer BE (1989) Laser angioplasty of iliac and femoropopliteal obstructive lesions. In: Höfling B, Pölnitz A v (eds) Interventional cardiology and angiology. Steinkopff, Darmstadt/Springer, Berlin Heidelberg New York, p 153

32. Höher M, Hombach V, Arnold G et al. (1987) High frequency recanalization of thrombotically occluded vessels in experimental pigs. Circulation 76 Suppl 4:IV–28
33. Dartsch PC, Bauriedel G, Höfling B, Betz (1989) Cell culture of human atheromatous plaque material. In: Höfling B, Pölnitz A v (eds) Interventional cardiology and angiology. Steinkopff, Darmstadt/Springer, Berlin Heidelberg New York, p 115
34. Palmaz JC, Richter GM, Nöldge G, Schatz GA, Robinson PD, Gardiner GA, Becker GJ, McLean GK, Denny DF, Lammer J, Paolini RM, Rees CR, Alvarado R, Heiss HW, Root HD, Rogers W (1988) Intraluminal stents in arteriosclerotic iliac artery stenosis: preliminary report of a multicenter study. Radiology 168:727
35. Schatz RA (1989) A view of vascular stents. Circulation 79:445
36. Simpson JB, Johnson DE, Thapliyal HV, Marks DS, Braden LJ (1985) Transluminal atherectomy: a new approach to the treatment of atherosclerotic vascular disease. Circulation 72: Suppl 2, III-146

## *Commentary*

*Bert Eikelboom*

There is no doubt that PTA has gained a definite and important place in the treatment of obstructive arterial disease. Initial scepticism and theoretical objections have disappeared because the technique has proved to be safe, effective and durable for suitable indications. As often occurs, the mechanism of the dilatation was found at a later stage. PTA has replaced vascular reconstructive surgery to a certain extent, mainly in the early stages of the disease where stenoses cause claudication. On the other hand, the impact of PTA for more severe limb ischaemia is, although fewer in number of procedures, more important from the clinical point of view. Most series on femoral and iliac PTA show that only 10–20% of all procedures are performed for rest pain and gangrene. How often this represented truly critical ischaemia is not known. Critical ischaemia is by definition characterized by the presence of extensive multilevel disease, which is less amenable to PTA than limited disease. There is an inverse relation between the success rate of PTA and the extent of the disease that has to be treated. This is no argument against PTA, because the same holds true for surgery. Both forms of treatment have also in common that the best results are obtained in the treatment of proximal lesions. The more distal one has to go, the poorer the results will be. Especially in patients with critical ischaemia, who are more ill than claudicants, it is of great importance to choose the procedure or sequence of procedures that causes the lowest morbidity and mortality. There are often many treatment options available: PTA alone, surgery alone, combined surgery and intra-operative PTA or PTA as initial treatment followed by surgery. Decision making is therefore a delicate process that requires a multi-disciplinary approach. Vascular surgeon, radiologist and angiologist all have to be aware of the possibilities and shortcomings of the various modes of treatment to allow the best treatment plan to be chosen in the individual patient.

The developments in thrombolytic therapy have made the need for a team approach even greater. The most difficult decision to make is in the patient who presents with acute on chronic ischaemia. The first question that arises here is whether there is enough time to try thrombolytic therapy before the ischaemia will cause irreversible damage to the leg. Clots may be extracted in conjunction with thrombolysis or lytic agents may be infused after surgical thrombectomy. In both instances, PTA may be necessary to treat the underlying cause of the thrombosis. If PTA is not feasible, bypass surgery offers an alternative. Similar strategies have to be followed when loss of limb is imminent because of an occluded bypass. Only specialized centres with good multidisciplinary teamwork will be able to make the right choices. Choices have to be made likewise with regard to recent technical innovations such as atherectomy, laser ablation and various rotating devices. Laser therapy creates only a narrow channel through an occluded segment and is therefore followed by balloon angioplasty to provide a wider lumen. The proper name for this procedure would therefore be "laser assisted balloon angioplasty". These techniques can be applied in the radiology suite or in the operating room. It is anticipated that more combinations of various treatment modalities will be seen and developments to improve radiology equipment in the operating room are under way. These include completely radiolucent operating tables and the advantages of DSA with improved real time images, roadmapping facilities and immediate playback. Intravascular ultrasound and angioscopy may be of further help in choosing the right procedure. The exact importance of all the various procedures that are available for clinical use at the moment is not yet known, because the field is changing so rapidly, which makes it difficult to perform proper evaluation of a certain technique.

What do we know exactly at the moment about the value of PTA for critical ischemia? Krings and Peters presented a good overview in this chapter. It shows that even for such a well-established method as PTA alone, it is difficult to define its exact place in patients other than claudicants. The number of this type of patient is small in most series and it is not always stated how many stenoses and occlusions were treated, how long the occlusions were and especially not what the status of the outflow vessels was. Not all series include the initial technical failure rate and technical success is not equivalent to clinical success. Long term results are often given only for initially successful cases, thereby creating an over-optimistic view. Proper lifetables should be constructed more often. It is because of these shortcomings in the literature that Krings and Peters have not tried to produce exact figures on the results of PTA in patients with critical ischaemia who have iliac or femoral stenoses or occlusions respectively. They rightfully state that results are 10–20% poorer than in stage II disease, which shows that the numbers that are given in the European Consensus Document are on the optimistic side. My own estimate from the literature is that technical and clinical success will be obtained in 75–80% in this particular type of patient. Newer types of catheters may expand indications for PTA to the infrapopliteal arteries, but no conclusions can be drawn at the moment on its efficiency in this area.

Some controversy exists on the role of angioplasty for aortic stenosis. There is the fear of embolization, but in our own experience PTA is very successful in this area and is therefore the method of choice. There is no doubt that PTA is preferred over surgery in iliac stenosis, but the choice is more difficult in the case of iliac occlusion and such factors as the length of occlusion, the presence of tortuosity, the quality of the contralateral artery, obesity and scarring in the groin, will have to be considered in making the right decision for an individual patient. Similar arguments can be given for femoro-popliteal disease.

Thrombolysis may revert long occlusions to short stenoses, which in turn may be treated more successfully by PTA. The concept of thrombolysis followed by PTA is therefore an attractive one. Local or low dose thrombolysis is preferred over systemic thrombolysis to reduce the risk of bleeding complications. It remains, however, a time-consuming technique, where further standardization on doses, methods and application is necessary. Full lysis will be achieved in some 60% of cases. The best indications in my view are recent acute on chronic occlusion, or recent bypass occlusion with critical ischaemia but no loss of sensory and motor function. A controversial indication is thrombosis of a popliteal aneurysm, a notoriously dangerous situation often followed by loss of limb. Surgical revascularization is not always possible. Thrombolysis is therefore considered by some to be a good solution, while others regard it a contraindication because of the danger of further embolization.

Krings and Peters point out that thrombolysis is not a harmless procedure. The risk of bleeding complications or embolization is considerable and more convincing early and long term results are needed before one can conclude that this type of therapy should be preferred over reconstructive surgery when that is technically possible. Although there seems to be general agreement that platelet aggregation inhibitors should be given to prevent thrombosis after peripheral PTA, it has to be pointed out that no proper controlled studies on this subject have been performed. It is not known how long adjunctive medical treatment should be given. On theoretical grounds it might be as good or even better to give anticoagulants. Other drugs that are potentially useful include low molecular weight heparin, thromboxane $A_2$ receptor blockers and prostanoids, but their clinical efficacy needs to be determined.

In conclusion, there is no doubt that PTA is an excellent technique that has become an important tool in the treatment of vascular disease. In true critical ischaemia, however, it is only occasionally an alternative to vascular surgery, because the extent of the disease is usually such that PTA is not feasible. Still, there is no doubt that it should be done whenever possible, to avoid the inherent risks of operation. Only close cooperation between the various specialists involved in this field will lead to the necessary discussion to make the right choice in an individual patient.

# Chapter 6

# Surgical Reconstruction for Critical Ischaemia

Peter Bell



## 6.1 Introduction

It has always been difficult to be certain of the results of surgical treatment for critical ischaemia, mainly because of the lack of a definition which would allow patients to be categorised appropriately [1]. Although Fontaine described his grading of limb ischaemia some years ago, there are patients, particularly in the Fontaine III Group who can improve spontaneously and may not fit the modern definition of critical ischaemia. Attempts have been made recently to define the R 2a
problem more clearly [2] and suggest that Fontaine III can be sub-divided into further Subgroups as explained earlier in this book. It should now be possible to carry out comparative studies to examine either surgical or other methods of treatment which will hopefully provide the data we need to decide which is the best method of treating the different causes of critical ischaemia. Precisely because of the lack of a definition most studies have, and continue to, contain a variety of patients who are said to be in danger of losing their limb or alternatively the reason for undertaking the procedure is not mentioned at all. The result is that many such patients have been suffering from claudication or are a group who would be expected to do well. Critical ischaemia therefore refers *only* to those patients who will, as far as we can tell, lose their leg if nothing is done to improve the circulation. Bearing this in mind the place of surgical reconstruction in critical ischaemia has to be examined objectively.

Prior to the advent of percutaneous techniques and in the absence of appropriate pharmacological therapy, surgery was the only method of treatment available for such patients. Now that other techniques are available we have to examine the place of surgery in critical ischaemia, bearing in mind that we are not discussing acute ischaemia where limb loss occurs in a relatively short period of time but chronic critical ischaemia which pursues a relentless course over a period of days or weeks.

The success of surgery depends very much on the level of the obstruction. As a general principle the more distal the obstruction the worse the results [3]. No one has defined what satisfactory limb salvage is but if we define it as a live patient with a viable limb at one year, bearing in mind that these are patients who have a mortality in the region of 30% at 5 years and 70% after 10 years [4], then one year patency rates are worth examining. As the site of the obstruction becomes more distal, the relationship between limb salvage and patency becomes less obvious. It is well known that limbs can remain viable even though a graft blocks after several months [5]. This is a well recognised phenomenon and does not mean that the graft was unnecessary. What often happens to patients who have critical ischaemia is that trauma to the foot results in infection, where the circulation is already relatively poor. If nothing is done, gangrene than supervenes and an amputation may become necessary. If a graft is done and if it stays patent for several months, the lesion can heal and the patient return to his previous state. Whether these patients have in the past satisfied the strict criteria for critical ischaemia remains to be elucidated in the future.

There is some evidence to suggest that the patency of short grafts is better than long conduits and this along with the better results to be expected from autologous vein has led to the use of multiple venous segments sutured between patent segments of artery [6], but there is no comparative evidence that this approach is better than with a long graft. At the time of writing this chapter there is no evidence that PTA is better or worse than surgical intervention for critical ischaemia, because of an absence in the literature of controlled comparative studies. A recent study comparing PTA and surgery for claudication suggested that PTA is associated with a lower mortality and produces results comparable with surgery [7]. Unfortunately however this study is of little relevance as such patients are not usually exposed to surgery and many can improve spontaneously.

## 6.2 Treatment of Choice for Specific Lesions

### 6.2.1 Aorto-Iliac Disease

Lesions in the aorta or iliac vessels do not often cause critical ischaemia on their
own but are usually part of a multilevel disease process; however, they can espe-
R 36 cially where embolisation is present. In these cases surgery can be expected to
produce excellent results with a patency at 1 year in excess of 95%. There is,
however, a price to pay with a mortality of approximately 5% in such patients. If
R 37 the patient is unfit for major abdominal surgery, however, then an alternative
procedure, such as an axillo-bifemoral graft for aorto-iliac obstruction, or a cross
over procedure for unilateral iliac obstruction can be used with good results [8].
Cross over grafts can be expected to show a patency rate in excess of 90% at one

year [9]. Axillo-bifemoral grafts on the other hand tend to do worse with a patency of about 70% at 1 year [10].

If the lesion is multi segmental then a bifurcated graft taken from the aorta to both femoral arteries without any attempt to deal with the distal obstruction will usually improve critical ischaemia sufficiently to allow limb salvage to take place. Obstructions of this type do not usually involve the renal arteries and the problem is due to atheroma of the aortic bifurcation. However, the aorta often blocks up to the level of the renal arteries but contains thrombus which can be easily removed. There is controversy as to whether an end to end or end to side anastomosis is best but end to side anastomoses are easier to perform and provide good results. The distal anastomosis should be placed across the mouth of the profunda femoris artery as this probably produces better long term results [11]. In patients with critical ischaemia a one year patency rate of more than 90% should be achieved with a 30 day mortality of less than 5% [8]. If the patient is not fit for surgery, alternative procedures should be considered, for example a retroperitoneal approach to the aorta allows the insertion of a bifurcated graft and is much less traumatic than a transperitoneal approach, with results which are equally good [12]. If the patient has a combination of aneurysmal and occlusive disease then surgery is of course mandatory.

If the patient is unfit for abdominal surgery, then an alternative technique such as an axillobifemoral graft should be considered. This method is not to be recommended however as a primary treatment, but can produce useful limb salvage in difficult patients who are elderly or unfit with low life expectancy. One year patency rates for such procedures are usually of the order of 65–70%.

If these grafts suddenly occlude then acute ischaemia can result. The best treatment is to unblock them with a combination of arterial strippers and Fogarty catheters [13]. Once they are unblocked the cause of the problem, which is usually an extension of the disease, can be dealt with by applying a vein patch to the outflow tract. Secondary patency rates can be enhanced in this way.

### 6.2.2 Iliac Disease

If a patient has a unilateral iliac occlusion which is greater than 5 or certainly R 40
10 cm in length, surgery is the treatment of choice if critical ischaemia is present
[8]. Once again it usually requires multisegment disease to cause ischaemia under
these circumstances. For obstructions less than 10 cm in length (Fig. 1) PTA can R 39
be effective. If, however, the proximal lesion is a stenosis of the iliac artery then
PTA gives excellent results [14].

For bilateral iliac occlusions, however, then either an aortic bifurcation graft or an extra anatomic procedure such as axillobifemoral grafting is the treatment of choice. In general PTA does not produce good results for occlusions of more than 5–10 cm in length [15] but controlled comparative trial data are lacking.

*Cross Over Graft*

This is an alternative to ilio-femoral grafting but the inflow of the donor limb must be checked before it is used. This can be done by using the papaverine test which involves measuring the pressure in the radial artery and femoral artery

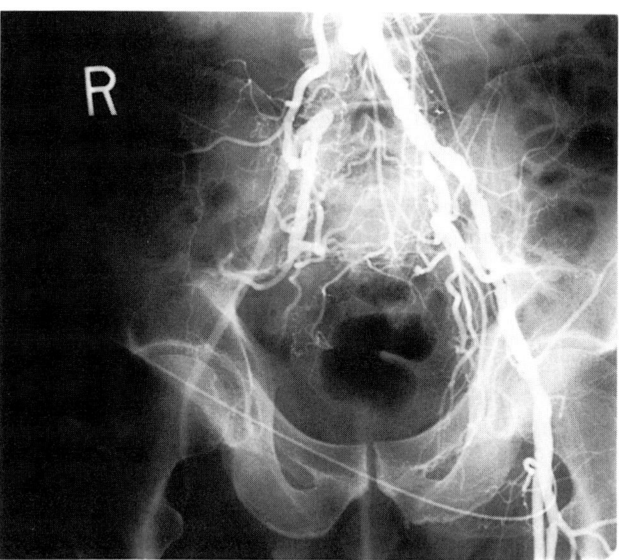


**Fig. 1.** Iliac occlusion which may be suitable for angioplasty

before and after giving the vasodilator papaverine. A fall of more than 15–20% in pressure suggests that an inflow problem is present [16]. This can be dealt with by angioplasty prior to using the vessel for a crossover donor site. If feasible, the iliac artery of the donor limb should be used as the donor vessel, routing the graft extra peritoneally to the operative side rather than using the femoral artery (Fig. 2). This allows easy access for angioplasty if this becomes necessary at a later date.

The results of cross over grafting are excellent with a one year patency rate in excess of 90% and a very low mortality [9]. The operation can be done under local anaesthesia. Complications can occur, including infection or steal of blood from the donor limb, but these are very rare.

### 6.2.3 Femoro-Popliteal Disease

R 41 Critical ischaemia due to occlusion of the femoral artery alone is rarely seen;
R 42 however, it is possible particularly if propagation of thrombus occurs or if there is embolisation. More usually the obstruction is multilevel and the proximal distal disease is associated with occlusions below the knee in the crural vessels. If the occlusion is causing critical ischaemia and, provided the obstruction is greater than 5–10 cm in length, some form of graft is the treatment of choice, particularly to the above knee popliteal artery if this proves possible. Alternatively an anastomosis to the below knee popliteal vessel can be performed. The conduit of choice for this procedure is the saphenous vein [17], either reversed or in situ as no differences has been found between these two procedures [18]. Artificial grafts such as PTFE either with or without extra luminal support and umbilical vein can be used successfully to the above or below knee popliteal artery with

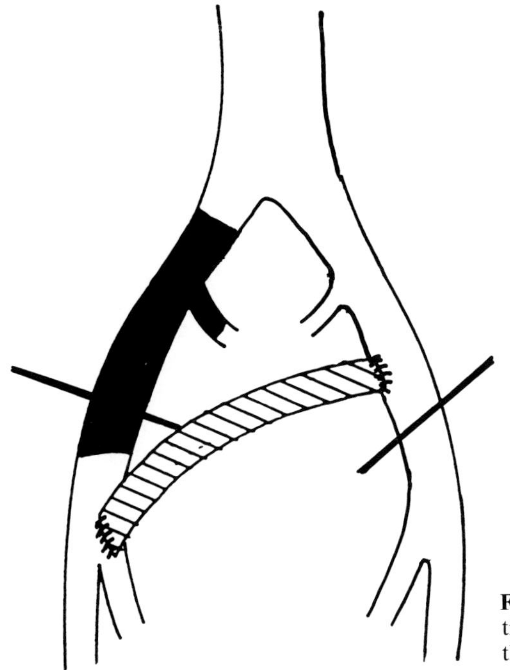

**Fig. 2.** Cross over graft for unilateral iliac obstruction. The donor site should be the iliac rather than the femoral artery

reasonable results [19]. With the exception of the above knee popliteal artery; artificial grafts should only be used if nothing else is available. The cephalic vein should be tried prior to using artificial grafts. Umbilical vein tends to become aneurysmal after several years and should not be used in younger patients in whom the life expectancy is reasonable. The results of femoro-popliteal grafting are good with two year patency rates in excess of 70%, particularly if vein is used [17].

*Occlusion of Femoro-Popliteal Grafts*

Grafts such as PTFE can be successfully unblocked but they usually occlude because of distal intimal hyperplasia and often need a revisional procedure to the outflow tract. Vein grafts are often impossible to unblock and the best treatment is thrombolysis using low dose Streptokinase or Urokinase delivered directly into the thrombus at a rate of 5000 units/hour following a test dose. This treatment is frequently successful and will lead to reopening of previously occluded vein grafts [20].

### 6.2.4 Femoro-Distal (Crural) Procedures

An increasing number of patients with critical ischaemia, especially the elderly, have occlusion of the proximal popliteal artery and a readily available crural vessel, either the peroneal or one of the tibials in the distal leg or foot. The results of R 43
surgery at this level are not as good as for proximal lesions with patency rates of

about 65–70% at one year for distal anastomoses if the vein is used [17]. With prosthetic materials taken to the ankle the patency rates are less than 25% [19,
R 44 20]. If such patients are operated on and for some reason the graft fails, the end result is either a higher amputation or a prolonged period of healing with a very poor wound. Quite apart from the question of success or failure, the increased cost of a failed vascular procedure, superimposed upon the other problems already mentioned, has to be borne in mind when making a decision [21]. The problem in such patients is deciding whether or not an operation is worthwhile, bearing in mind the high mortality and, as already mentioned, a reasonable expectancy of saving the limb for one year would be acceptable. In those cases where salvage is virtually impossible then the question of a primary amputation must be borne in mind. Current research is trying to define those patients who would not respond to an operation and in whom the chances of success are so small that a primary amputation is the best treatment. Other temporary measures such as PTA have not as yet produced good results in patients with a distal occlusion and a poor run off.

In such patients preoperative arteriography is frequently of little use (Fig. 3); if no vessels are seen in the lower leg, it does not mean none are there. The same criticism would apply to intravenous DSA. Consequently other methods have to be used to try and find a patent artery at the ankle or mid calf. This can be done by listening for a Doppler signal over all three crural vessels at the ankle with the legs hanging over the side of the couch, when a signal indicating a patent vessel

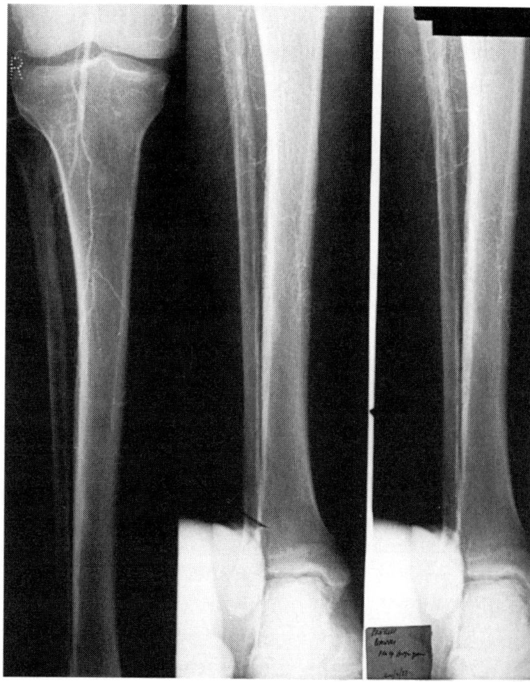

**Fig. 3.** Preoperative angiogram showing no vessels in the lower limb. This does not mean that all vessels are occluded

can be heard. A new technique termed pressure generated run off (P.G.R.) has recently been described [22]. This involves placing a cuff around the lower thigh and upper calf of the patient and applying a rapid intermittent pressure. By listening over each vessel in turn, a signal can be heard and a pulse wave seen. A signal means continuity between the origin of the artery and the cuff (Fig. 4). If

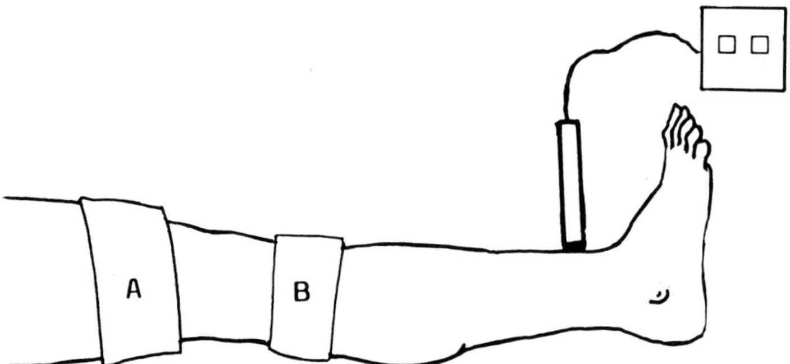


**Fig. 4.** Cuff A applied just above the knee – Cuff B inflated intermittently by compressed air to produce a signal which is listened for at the ankle with a Doppler probe

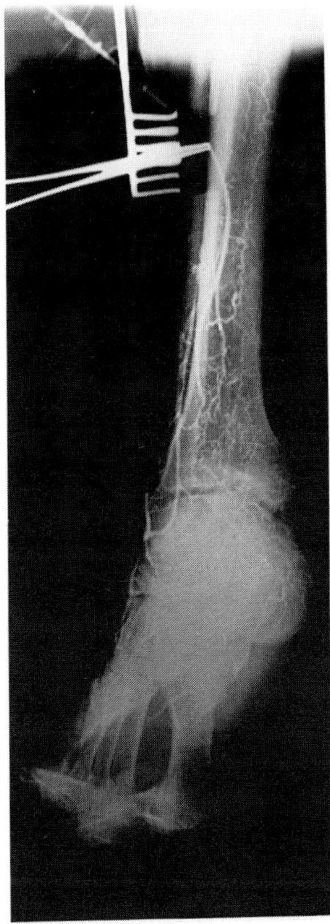

**Fig. 5.** On table angiogram (same patients as Fig. 3) showing a good peroneal artery (approached after removing a segment of fibula) with a good run off into the foot

no signal is found, the possibility must exist that there are blocked arteries in the foot. Once an appropriate artery has been selected the vessel must be explored and contrast injected on table to produce an angiogram (Fig. 5). If this confirms a reasonable vessel with outflow into the plantar arch the operation can proceed, after an attempt has been made to assess the likely end result. This can be done by perfusing a fixed volume of blood at constant flow down the distal artery in order to measure peripheral resistance.

Evidence is now accumulating that a high peripheral resistance will lead to early graft failure and that primary amputation may be the best option [23]. There is controversy about this suggestion and more objective evidence of success or failure has to be obtained before individual patients can be treated in this way. If the resistance is high then the likelihood is that an amputation would be best for that patient. Grafts to the crural vessels should use the long saphenous vein, if at all possible, and the in situ technique will give the best results [19]. Artificial grafts to the lower calf or ankle do not generally do well. If the resistance is low then vein graft has a good chance of succeeding. Following the insertion of a piece of vein graft attempts should be made to measure the resistance and flow in order to assess whether there are technical problems. A completion angiogram is an alternative, but some technique should be used to assess the operation before closing the wound. If the pre-reconstruction resistance is high, the possibility of including an arteriovenous fistula at the distal anastomosis, to allow an increased flow through the graft and maintain patency, should be considered although there is no evidence at the present time that this does any good [24].

### R 38 6.2.5 Multisegment Disease

Very often critical ischaemia is due to disease occurring at two levels, that is aortoiliac plus femoral popliteal or distal. In this situation there is still some controversy as to what should be done. However, it is fairly clear that if the proximal lesion is dealt with then the distal lesion does not need immediate attention [25], although there are papers which suggest that both should be dealt with in the first instance [26]. When obstructions occur more distally they are usually a combination of femoropopliteal and crural disease and the results are worse. Prosthetics can be used for the upper crural vessels and if some form of vein cuff is interposed between the vein and the graft, the results are probably better [27, 28]. Beyond the mid calf level however the vein alone is recommended in the in situ position and patency rates of 60–70% can be expected for crural vessels at 1 year [17]. If prosthetic material is used below this point then the results are very poor with patency rates at one year of about 20% [29]. The mortality for these patients who are usually frail and have other diseases is high, although if spinal or local anaesthesia is used this can be reduced. A further requirement for surgical reconstruction is that the patient should be fit enough for the procedure and that run off should be reasonable. Defining what is reasonable has so far been difficult but evidence is now appearing in the literature to suggest that the peripheral resistance measured either during or before surgery can give a clue to the likely outcome [30]. Patients with a high peripheral resistance and distal disease are probably not worth reconstructing and the possibility of primary amputation as discussed later in this book should be considered [23]. A reconstructive procedure should only be attempted if there is a reasonable chance of saving a useful limb, particularly as there is a disadvantage in that early graft failure may worsen the ischaemia and result in an amputation at a higher level [31] and an increased mortality [31]. Quite apart from these problems, the question of audit and cost has to be considered and a failed procedure undoubtedly increases the overall costs [21]. For these reasons some lesions may be best dealt with by PTA or thrombolysis as discussed earlier.

## 6.3 Graft Surveillance and Occlusion R 22

*Graft Surveillance*

It has been shown that in the first year following surgery, stenoses develop in vein grafts or intimal hyperplasia in prosthetic grafts causing premature occlusion in as many as 20% of cases [32]. Such stenoses (Fig. 6), when they occur, can be dealt with by angioplasty or by revisional surgery. This means that every graft inserted has to be examined on a regular basis if this is to be avoided.

The best method of looking for graft stenosis is either duplex scanning, which can detect a stenosis by detecting an increase in the peak flow or DSA which can

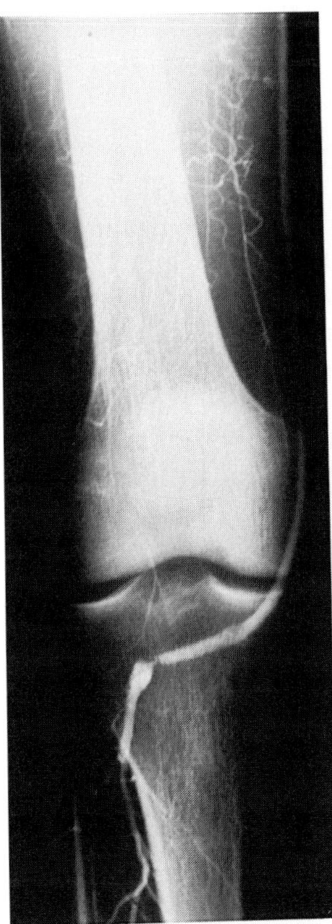

**Fig. 6.** An example of a stenosis at the lower end of a vein graft detected by duplex scanning

provide good results but is invasive. If a stenosis is discovered the patient must be dealt with quickly by angioplasty or surgery, otherwise the graft will thrombose and be lost; once a vein graft has thrombosed it cannot be easily salvaged, except perhaps by the use of thrombolytic agents.

If the graft fails quickly (within 24 hours) it should not be explored unless there is a reasonable chance of a successful outcome. For example, in a patient with a very high resistance found at the original operation, the chances of successful restoration of flow are poor and amputation may be the better option. Graft occlusion can also be reduced if grafts, particularly vein grafts, are examined regularly by some method in the first year following their insertion. The nature of graft failure remains obscure, but stenoses which occur either at the anastomosis or along the course of the vein are often fibrous in nature. Such stenoses are most easily seen by non-invasive methods such as duplex; DSA is also useful but invasive. Stenoses can occur in as many as 20% of vein grafts in the first year but do not seem to occur later. If they do occur, then angiography will confirm their presence and they can be dealt with either by angioplasty or surgery. In this way patency rates can be improved further. The question of when a primary amputation should be done remains controversial; if there is a reasonable chance of limb salvage (although some would say any chance of limb salvage), then a reopening procedure should be attempted. It is very important to stress that in no patient should an amputation be performed until every effort is made to ensure that a reconstructive procedure is not possible. This is usually by means of preoperative angiography.

## 6.4 Sympathectomy

Surgical sympathectomy was a common and popular method of dealing with critical ischaemia but there is no evidence that this technique has any value for such patients [33]. An occasional patient may benefit but there is no way of forcasting which one might do so, with the exception of thromboangiitis obliterans, where a sympathectomy may as a general rule give reasonable results. The possibility of using a chemical sympathectomy with phenol should be borne in mind as there is some evidence that this treatment will alleviate pain without necessarily increasing flow in patients with critical ischaemia. A patient with stable rest pain whose only problem is pain without progressive ischaemia can be helped by this technique and it should be considered [34].

## 6.5 Summary

*The consensus view*

R 21 From what has been said above, it is clear that provided there is a reasonable run off and the patient is fit for the procedure, surgical treatment will provide excellent longterm results. Most surgeons would agree that stenoses or short obstructions of up to 5 cm can often be dealt with by percutaneous transluminal angioplasty, although comparative trials of this treatment remain to be assessed and critical ischaemia is rarely caused by short lesions, except in multisegment disease. For more distal obstructions the chances of success diminish, with most graft losses occurring in the first three months following surgery. Attempts must be made to ensure that the operation has been done properly, particularly with procedures below the inguinal ligament and graft patency should be confirmed in some way at the end of surgery by either angiography, flow or resistance measurements.

Because surgery produces excellent results in proximal occlusions, it should be used in this situation in appropriate patients. If the aorta or iliac vessels are stenosed then PTA is the treatment of choice. Occlusions greater than 5 cm in length do relatively badly with PTA and surgery should be used for them. Either bifurcation grafting, ilio-femoral procedures, cross over grafting or axillo-femoral grafts should be undertaken and the results are good. If embolisation is occurring, then clearly surgery must be undertaken to prevent the lesion getting worse. For long occlusions in the femoropopliteal arteries grafting is the procedure of choice, and PTA has not as yet been shown to produce comparable results in such patients with critical ischaemia, although laser assistance thrombolysis and atherectomy may improve the results in the long term. If possible vein should be used as results are better, particularly below the knee. In general, prosthetic grafts to ankle vessels rarely succeed but they might allow an alternative to amputation, especially in those patients where healing of a lesion leads to preservation of the limb.

## References


1. Bell PRF, Charlesworth D, De Palma R, Jamieson C (1982) The definition of critical ischaemia of a limb. Br J Surg 69:52.1
2. Wolfe JHN (1988) Critical ischaemia – is this concept of value? In: Greenhalgh RW, Jamieson CW, Nicolaides AN (eds) Limb salvage and amputation for vascular disease. WB, Saunders, London, pp 3–10
3. Bell PRF (1985) Are distal vascular procedures worthwhile? Br J Surg 335:72
4. Dormandy JA, Mahir MS (1986) The natural history of peripheral atheromatous disease of the legs. In: Greenhalgh, Jamieson, Nicolaides (eds) Vascular surgery: issues in current practice. Grune and Stratton, London, pp 3–19
5. Dardik H, Miller N, Dardik A, Ibrahim IM, Susman B, Berry SM, Wolodiger F, Kahn M, Dardik I (1988) A decade of experience with the gluteraldehyde tanned human umbilical cord vein graft for revascularisation of the a lower limb. J Vasc Surg 7:336–346
6. Ascer E, Veith FJ, Gupta SK, White SA, Curtis MA, Bakal W, Wengerter K, Sprayregen S (1988) Short vein grafts: a superior option for arterial reconstructions to poor or compromised outflow tracts. J Vasc Surg 7:370–378
7. Wilson SE, Wolf GL, Cross A (1989) Percutaneous transluminal angioplasty versus operation for peripheral arteriosclerosis. Report of a randomised trial in a selected group of patients. J Vasc Surg 9:1–9
8. Piotrowski J, Pearce WH, Bell R, Patt Anita, Rutherford R (1986) Aortofemoral bypass: the operation of choice for unilateral iliac ischaemia? J Vasc Surg 8:211–218
9. Fahal AH, McDonald AM, Marston A (1989) Femoro-femoral bypass in unilateral iliac artery occlusion. Br J Surg 76:22–25
10. Corbett RR, Taylor PR, Chilvers A et al. (1984) Axillo femoral bypass grafts in poor risk patients with critical ischaemia. Ann Roy Coll Surg Eng 66:170–173

11. Brewster DC (1984) Aortoiliac occlusive disease. Bell PRF, Tilney N (eds) Vascular surgery. Butterworth, London, pp 78–107
12. Johnson JN, McLoughlin GA, Wake PN, Helsoby PR (1986) Comparison of extra peritoneal and trans peritoneal methods of aortoiliac reconstruction: twenty years experience. J Cardiovasc Surg 27:561–565
13. Macpherson DS, Bell PRF (1982) The unblocking of occluded dacron grafts. In: Greenhalg R (ed) Extra anatomic and secondary arterial reconstruction. Pitman, London, pp 334–345
14. Morris JF, Wayne-Johnson K, Rae M (1986) Improvement after successful percutaneous dilatation treatment of occlusive peripheral arterial disease. Surg Gynaecol Obstet 163:453–457
15. Murie JA (1988) Percutaneous transluminal angioplasty and vascular surgery for lower limb ischaemia. Br J Surg 75:1051–1053
16. Quin RO, Evans DH, Bell PRF (1975) Haemodynamic assessment of the aortoiliac segment. J Cardiovasc Surg 16:586–589
17. Rutherford RB, Jones DN, Bergentz SE, Bergqvist D, Comerota A, Dardik H, Fliu WH, Fry WJ, McIntyre K, Moore WS, Shah DM, Yano T (1988) Factors affecting the patency of infra inguinal bypass. J Vasc Surg 8:236–246
18. Watelet J, Chacysson E, Poels D, Menhard JF, Papion H, Testart SN (1986) In situ versus reversed saphenous vein for femoropopliteal bypass: a prospective randomised study of 100 cases. Ann Vasc Surg 1:441–452
19. Sterpetti AW, Schultz RD, Feldhaus RJ, Peetz DJ Jr (1988) Seven year experience with polyetrafluorethylene as above knee femoropopliteal bypass graft: is it worthwhile to preserve the autologous saphenous vein? J Vasc Surg 8:229–235
20. Gardener GA Jr, Harrington DP, Koltrun W, Whittemore A, Mannick JA, Levin DC (1987) Salvage of occluded arterial bypass grafts by means of thrombolysis. J Vasc Surg 9:426–432
21. Gupta SK, Veith FJ, Ascer E, White Flores SA, Gleedman ML (1988) Cost factors in limb threatening ischaemia due to infrainguinal arthersclerosis. European J Vasc Surg 2:151–155
22. Beard JD, Scott JA, Evans JM, Skidmore R, Horrocks M (1988) Pulse generated run off: a new method of determining calf vessel patency. Br J Surg 75:361–363
23. Parvin SD, Evans DH, Bell PRF (1985) Peripheral resistance measurement in the assessment of severe peripheral vascular disease. Br J Surg 72:751–753
24. Harris PL, Campbell H (1983) Adjuvant distal arterio-venous shunt with femorotibial bypass for critical ischaemia. Br J Surg 70:377–379
25. Harris PL (1987) Management of combined segment disease. European J Vasc Surg 1:367–369
26. Charles D (1987) Problems related to run in and run off with reference to the profundafemoris artery and secondary femoropopliteal bypass. Acta Chir Scand 538–543
27. Miller JH, Foreman RK, Ferguson L, Faris I (1984) Interposition vein cuff for anastomosis of prosthesis to small artery. Aust and New Zeal J Surg 54:283–286
28. Taylor RS, McFarland RJ, Cox MI (1987) An investigation into the causes of failure of PTFE grafts. European J Vasc Surg 1:335–345
29. Klimach O, Underwood CJ, Charlesworth D (1984) Femoropopliteal bypass with a Goretex prosthesis: a long term follow up. Br J Surg 71:821–824
30. Ascer E, Veith FJ, Morris L, Lesser ML, Gupta SK, Samson RH, Scher VA, White-Flores SA (1984) Components of outflow resistance and their correlation with graft patency of lower extremity arterial reconstructions. J Vasc Surg 1:817–828
31. Dardik H, Kahn M, Dardik I, Sussman B, Ibrahim IM (1982) Influence of failed vascular bypass procedures on conversion of below knee to above knee amputation levels. Surgery 91:64–69
32. Wolfe JHN, Macpherson GAD (1987) The failing femoro distal graft. European J Vasc Surg 1:295–297
33. Campbell WB (1988) Sympathectomy for chronic arterial ischaemia. European J Vasc Surg 2:357–364
34. Cross FW, Cotton LT (1985) Chemical lumbar sympathectomy for ischaemic rest pain. Am J Surg 150:341–345

## *Commentary*

*Heinz Heidrich*

There is no doubt that Professor Bell's very practical strategy for the surgical treatment of patients with critical limb ischaemia is both comprehensive and practical. He presents a very balanced surgical approach which should receive wide acceptance. Perhaps, however, it does not fully take into account the rapid recent developments in the non-surgical therapy of these patients which could be expanded into a more integrated combined medical and surgical approach. Despite the difficulty of evaluating the newer medical therapies, it is time now to begin to integrate the two approaches and to avoid perpetuating an increasingly artifical separation.

Placebo-controlled prospective clinical trials have shown therapeutic efficacy of pentoxyfylline, naftidrofuryl and buflomedil in intermittent claudication (Fontaine stage II). However such double blind studies, showing a therapeutic benefit in critical limb ischaemia with systolic ankle pressures below 50 mm Hg or a $tcPO_2$ of less than 20 mm Hg, are not yet available for these conventional vasoactive drugs. The reason is that such trials have not been undertaken, rather than established evidence of inefficacy in such trials. So far there have been only very small and methodologically flawed clinical studies of such drugs, where both positive and negative results can be discounted. But even a critical reviewer has to admit that some of these drugs, usually given orally, can be effective in critical limb ischaemia when administered intravenously or intra-arterially. We have retrospectively analysed 697 patients with Fontaine stage III and IV disease, who have fulfilled partly the criteria for critical limb ischaemia proposed in the Consensus Document. The relief of rest pain was observed after treatment with naftidrofuryl (n=119) in 51.9 percent and after pentoxyfylline (n=221) in 50 percent of cases. In 154 patients given prostanoids, 62.7% became free of rest pain. This can be compared with primary catheter dilatation in 62 patients where 62.7% were improved to Fontaine stage I or II disease. Selective catheter lysis (n=42) showed similar improvement in 42.1% of cases and primary vascular surgery (n=176) in 71.2% of cases. Whilst it is accepted that such preliminary retrospective analyses are not stringent enough to allow the proposal of definite therapeutic recommendations, they should encourage further attempts at large prospective studies to establish the possible therapeutic role of these medications in the treatment of critical limb ischaemia.

The use of prostanoids represents one of the newer treatment modalities, where large scale but open studies in Fontaine stage III and IV as well as some controlled studies using it either intra-arterially or intravenously suggest that rest pain and necroses were reduced or disappeared. In our large but uncontrolled study, mean treatment period of 27.1 days, rest pain was completely relieved in 27.8% and improved to a clinically relevant degree in 40.1%. After a mean of 21.9 months, 66% of patients who had lost their rest pain during prostanoid treatment were still pain free and without tissue necrosis. It is interesting that this result is comparable to the long term results following reconstructive surgery as described by Bell. Similar favourable results appear to be achievable with prostanoids.

This development of pharmacological therapies, combined with catheter reopening procedures, can be used to complement and complete Bell's surgical strategy. The following additional and alternative recommendations would result in a more complete surgical and medical strategy:

1. Some patients with short or long arterial occlusions of the aorto-iliac region are unsuitable for reconstructive surgery or PTA because they are too high a risk or refuse consent for any form of interventional treatment. In some of these cases, systemic thrombolysis should be considered, as this can be successful even with longer obstructions, provided it is not older than 6 to 12 months and peripheral rest pain or necrosis are relatively recent. Treatment with vasoactive drugs or prostanoids is not effective in critical limb ischaemia due to aorto-iliac occlusions.

2. In patients with isolated occlusions of the popliteal or crural arteries, or a combination of femoral and crural artery occlusions where surgery may be unsuccessful or dangerous, intra-arterial or intravenous prostanoids should be the primary treatment. Only patients who do not respond to this therapy, or whose ankle systolic pressure is near zero and have a $tcPO_2$ of less than 10 to 20 mm Hg, should be considered for vascular reconstruction as a primary form of therapy. It is not known at present if the effectiveness of prostanoid treatment depends on the length of the occluded segment.

3. Prostanoids are the treatment of first choice when critical limb ischaemia is not improved following reopening of the aorto-iliac segment, because of more distal occlusions.

4. Prostanoids are the treatment of choice in thromboangitis obliterans. Sympathectomy in this condition has not been shown to be effective and catheter reopening procedures or vascular reconstructions are only indicated as an absolutely last resort for limb salvage.

The practical surgical strategies proposed by Bell are optimal but need to be integrated with newer medical modalities. This also applies to his highly critical cost-oriented position to primary amputation versus repeated attempts at reconstruction of femoro-popliteal occlusions. There nevertheless remains much more clinical work which needs to be carried out to delineate the exact role of the different forms of therapy for the treatment of critical limb ischaemia. This requires stringent comparative studies in which diagnostic classification has to be based on the criteria of critical limb ischaemia as formulated in the Consensus Document. The surgical and catheter procedures have to be subjected to the same hard analysis used for assessing medical therapies. In all probability, only an efficient interdisciplinary cooperative effort by vascular surgeons, angiologists and interventional radiologists can achieve the best possible results in patients with critical limb ischaemia.

# Chapter 7

# Amputations

Peter Harris and Paul Moody



## 7.1 Introduction

Major amputation of the leg is a destructive operation which represents a crude but sometimes necessary approach to the problem of critical ischaemia. It is a procedure which is tolerated poorly with a hospital mortality of up to 30 per cent and a high incidence of non-fatal complications often necessitating a prolonged stay in hospital [1]. Even after intensive rehabilitation aided by sophisticated modern prostheses satisfactory mobility is achieved in considerably less than half of the patients [2]. The effect of this surgery and its consequences on elderly, frail individuals can be totally demoralising. Two years after operation approximately 40 per cent will have died and of the survivors many will have become heavily dependant upon family, friends or the state [2]. To add to their burdens at least 30 per cent will develop critical ischaemia of their other leg before the die [1].

Amputation, therefore, is an undertaking which is extremely costly not only financially but also in terms of human suffering and it must be a primary responsibility of vascular specialists to reduce the necessity for it to a minimum. Taking this premise as a starting point the European Working Group set out to define in general terms the place of primary amputation in the management of critical ischaemia and its recommendations form the basis of this chapter.

## 7.2 Incidence of Major Amputations for Vascular Disease

In 1986 a total of 5,780 new patients were referred to limb fitting centres in England, Wales and Northern Ireland, 64 per cent of whom had had major

**Table 1.** Aetiology of amputation in 1986. (Only those referred to limb fitting centres in Great Britain)

| | Male | Female | Total | Percentage |
|---|---|---|---|---|
| Vascular | 2434 | 1262 | 3696 | 63.9 |
| Diabetes | 765 | 391 | 1156 | 20.0 |
| Trauma | 422 | 105 | 527 | 9.1 |
| Malignancy | 122 | 98 | 220 | 3.8 |
| Infection | 72 | 37 | 109 | 1.9 |
| Deformity | 46 | 26 | 72 | 1.3 |
| Total | 3861 | 1919 | 5780 | 100.0 |

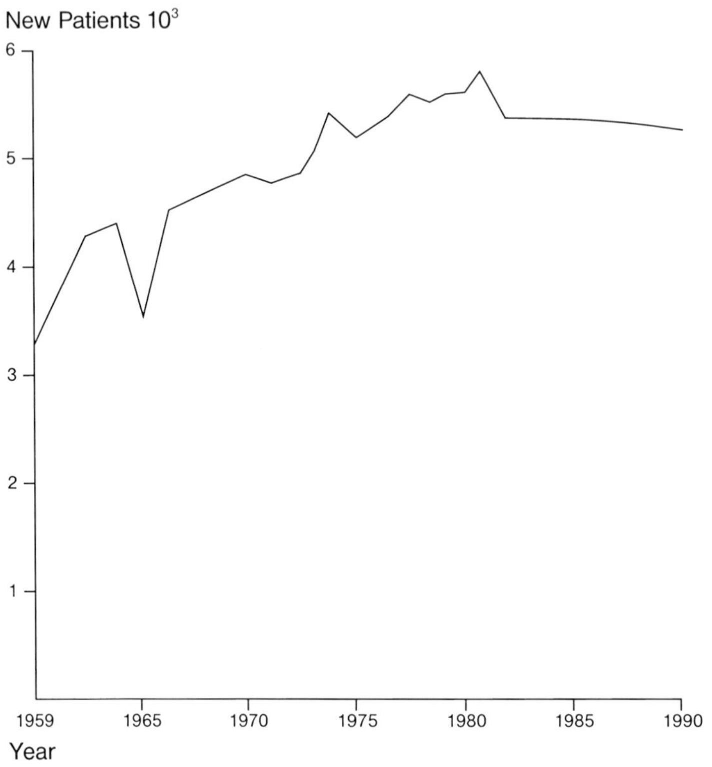


**Fig. 1.** The total number of new patients attending limb fitting centres in England, Wales and Northern Ireland 1959–1985

amputations for vascular disease and another 20 per cent for complications of diabetes [1] (Table 1).

Since may amputees, particularly those with widespread chronic arterial disease are not referred for an artificial limb, it has been estimated that these statistics could underestimate the true incidence of amputation for vascular insufficiency by up to 50 per cent. The incidence of amputation for critical ischaemia in the general population of the British Isles is therefore probably between 10 and 15 per 100000 per annum and similar rates are likely for most other European countries. Taking new attendances at limb fitting centres in Britain as a guide between the years 1960 to 1979 the number of major amputations increased at a rate of about 3 per cent per annum, but the incidence appears to have levelled off during the last decade [1] (Fig. 1).

More detailed analysis of the available data shows that the amputation rate in those over 80 years has increased by approximately 4 per cent over the whole decade, while that for the age group 60–79 years has decreased by 1.2 per cent [1]. During the same period the population aged over 60 years has increased by nearly 10 per cent and there are therefore now considerably fewer amputations being carried out relative to the population at risk than there were 10 years ago. This is the first hopeful sign that preventive measures including reconstructive arterial intervention in its various forms are beginning to have a significant impact on the natural history of this disease.

In patients with intermittent claudication the long term risk of amputation is surprisingly low at only 1.6 per cent and 1.8 per cent in two large epidemiological studies [3, 4]. However, in a recent multicentre investigation of critical ischaemia the amputation rate was 19 per cent at the first admission with a further 25 per cent having major amputations inside the first twelve months [5].

More aggressive treatment of claudicants, by angioplasty for example, may effect a reduction in amputation rates in time, but for the present, the most realistic chance of reducing further the need for amputation is to ensure optimal management of those with already established critical ischaemia.

## 7.3 Indications for Primary Amputation in Critical Ischaemia

Recommendation 25 of the Critical Ischaemia Consensus Document states that "Primary amputation should only be undertaken if the possibility of revascularisation procedures has been excluded". This statement places emphasis on the need to consider all other alternatives first and the implication is that the decision to offer amputation should be reached only by a carefully considered process of elimination. In practice revascularisation might be rejected because it is deemed to be inappropriate, unsafe, impossible or inadvisable (Table 2). R 25

There can be little dispute about the need for amputation in those who, through reasons of neglect, do not present until they have developed irreversible

**Table 2.** Some Reasons for Rejecting Attempts at Revascularisation

| | |
|---|---|
| Reconstruction inappropriate | Necrosis of a major part of the limb<br>Functionally useless limb |
| Reconstruction unsafe | Life threatening toxaemia from ischaemic tissue |
| Reconstruction impossible | Complete absence of operable distal vessels |
| Reconstruction inadvisable | Patent distal vessels and revascularisation technically possible but with poor chance of success |

necrosis in a major part of the limb, those whose lives are seriously threatened by toxaemia from muscle necrosis or those in whom critical ischaemia develops in a limb which has already been rendered useless by some other cause. The Consensus Document advises that angiography should always be performed before major amputation is undertaken but patients in these categories might be considered exceptions.

Far more problematical is the patient with a viable and potentially useful limb. In order to make the best decision for these individuals, detailed information is required about the distribution and effect of the arterial disease in the limb.

## 7.4 Investigation of Patients Prior to Major Amputation

The Working Group decided that angiography should always be performed before major amputation. However, it must be emphasised that pre-operative radiology represents a minimal requirement only. In a great majority of patients the feasibility of revascularisation is determined by the presence or absence of patent distal vessels. It is well recognised that in the presence of extensive proximal occlusions pre-operative angiography even with digital enhancement of the images can fail to demonstrate poorly perfused but patent distal arteries. For this reason standard angiographic techniques on their own are unreliable indicators of operability and are therefore an insecure basis upon which to make a decision for amputation.

Direct surgical exploration of the vessels at the ankle supplemented by on-table angiography is the most certain way of assessing the situation accurately [6, 7] but has obvious disadvantages.

Recently a simple method has been described for detecting patent vessels pre-operatively with Doppler ultrasound [7]. A pulse is generated by rapid inflation of a pneumatic cuff placed around the calf and this can be detected distally with a Doppler probe in any vessel which is patent. If its reliability is confirmed, this technique of pulse generated run-off assessment (P.G.R.) could substantially reduce the need for "blind" surgical exploration.

Patency of a vessel distal to an occlusion does not by itself make revascularisation a feasible proposition. It is necessary to know also something about the quality of the vessel and its potential capacity to receive and distribute to the ischaemic tissue an adequate supply of blood – that is the run-off. It is often possible to gain some impression about these factors from pre-operative X-rays and from P.G.R. but on-table angiography gives much more accurate information about the pedal circulation and the most suitable vessel to use for any proposed reconstruction [9].

It is possible also to assess objectively the capacity of the run-off from intra-operative measurements of resistance or impedance, from which deductions can be made about the relative chances of any reconstruction which is under consideration being successful [10, 11]. While measurements of this type are still experimental and therefore not widely available, both pre-operative and intra-operative angiography are essential pre-requisites before the feasibility of distal reconstruction can be eliminated with certainty and both of these investigations should ideally be undertaken before a potentially useful limb is amputated.

## 7.5 Limb Salvage Reconstruction Versus Primary Amputation

A most difficult situation to judge to the patient's best advantage is that in which surgical reconstruction may be technically possible, but with a poor chance of lasting success. This most often occurs when occlusive disease extends into the infracrural vessels as is often the case in those with critical ischaemia. Although bypass grafts to the ankle and foot are now commonplace, some of these operations are approaching the limits of surgical efficacy. Autologous vein grafts from groin to ankle provide at least an even chance of limb salvage and are indicated wherever possible, but the results from synthetic grafts in this situation fall considerably short of this with patency rates at one year of only 25 to 30 per cent [12]. Given the necessity for a long bypass and the non-availability of sufficient autologous vein, a decision must be made whether to attempt reconstruction or to advise primary amputation. There are those who would always recommend reconstruction on the grounds that amputation so disadvantages the patient that attempted revascularisation has everything to gain and nothing to lose. This approach would not be contentious if there were not a price to be paid for failure, but a limb which is marginally critical can be made worse, and amputation following a failed reconstruction may have to be made at a higher level than would otherwise have been the case and this could be disastrous for the patient, if it involves conversion of a below knee stump to one above the knee. Account must be taken also of the risks of surgery, including death, which at best are additive and at worst multiplied when amputation follows rapidly after an unsuccessful bypass. An elderly arteriosclerotic patient who has sequential operations within a short space of time is in serious danger of his life. On the other hand if all patients in this category were to be offered only primary amputation, some at least would be denied the very considerable advantages of a successful revascularisation. It is tempting to try to specify those operations with expected patency rates above and below a minimal limit judged to represent a worthwhile measure of success. However, attempts to do so encounter several difficulties. Firstly, there is considerable lack of agreement amongst experts concerning the definition of "a worthwhile measure of success". Secondly, there is considerable variation in the results of the same operation from centre to centre, and thirdly, there is considerable variation in the level of fitness and mental attitude between individual patients, and what would be reasonable for one would be totally unreasonable for another. Therefore, firm recommendations in this connection are not possible and a more flexible approach is required.

The Working Group made the observation that "In some cases primary amputation may be better than subjecting the patient to repeated surgical procedures with little chance of success and increasing mortality and morbidity. This can be a very difficult decision where a team approach may be particularly useful." Recommendation 44 states that "Prosthetic grafts to the ankle vessels or R 44
below rarely succeed, however, they might still be indicated as an alternative to amputation". Each case should therefore be assessed on its individual merits but a most important guide to the decision making process is the surgeon's own "track-record" for each of the operative procedures under consideration, and it is therefore an essential requirement for all those involved in this type of work to maintain an accurate audit of their results.

## 7.6 Level of Major Amputations and Rehabilitation

Below knee amputations have considerable advantages over above knee amputations with an average operative mortality rate of about 8 per cent compared to 18 per cent and satisfactory rehabilitation with a prosthesis in the order of 50 per cent as opposed to 25 per cent [13]. In fact patients requiring below knee and above knee amputations are not directly comparable and the difference in mortality is most unlikely to be accounted for solely by the level of the operation. However, the principal advantage of the below knee procedure is related to preservation of the natural knee joint which can certainly make an enormous difference to the degree of mobility which patients are likely to achieve following fitting of their prosthetic limb. Despite this, above knee operations still account for 49.2 per cent and those below the knee only 46 per cent of the total number of major lower limb amputations in the United Kingdom [1]. It is now well recognised that this ratio can and should be reversed, indeed some centres have been able to achieve below knee amputation rates of 70–80 per cent [14]. There are indications of a general trend towards relatively more below knee amputations during the last 10 years [1] (Fig. 2) but this trend could probably be accelerated to the considerable advantage of many patients.

The disadvantage of below knee amputations is that they have poorer healing rates and a greater need for revisional surgery than above knee amputations. On

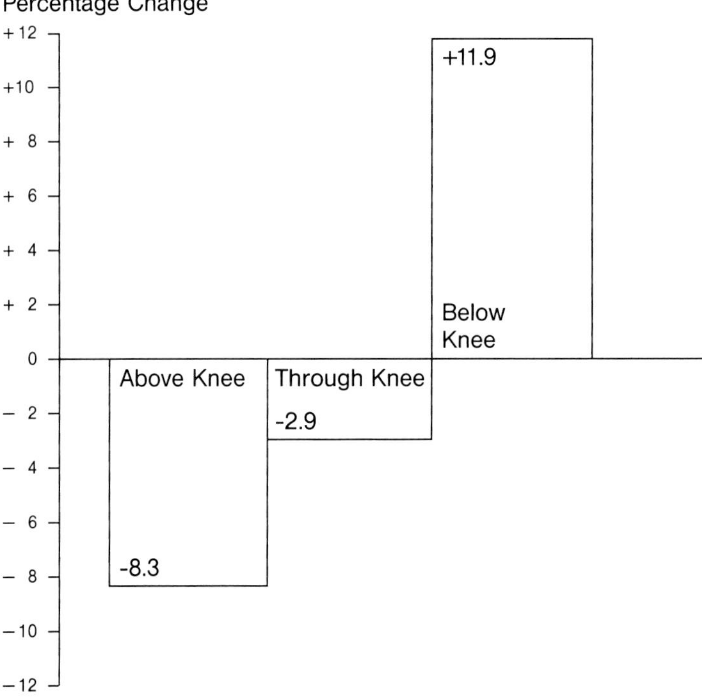


**Fig. 2.** Percentage change in above knee, through-knee and below knee amputations in England, Wales and Northern Ireland 1976–1986

average 70 per cent can be expected to heal primarily and another 15 per cent by secondary intention, but the remaining 15 per cent will require conversion to an above knee amputation [13]. Optimism that the skewflap technique of below knee amputation might be associated with a better healing rate than the conventional long posterior flap operation has not been borne out by a recent randomised study [15]. Unfortunately an anticipated failure rate in the order of 15 per cent is sufficient to dissuade some surgeons from using the below knee procedure as their preferred operation.

The essential pre-requisite for a successful below knee amputation, apart from a good range of movement in the knee joint, is skin perfusion at mid calf level which is adequate to permit healing of a surgical wound. The currently high failure rate is an indication that clinical assessment of this, even in experienced hands, is very unreliable. Evidence is now accumulating that the application of objective measurements of skin perfusion not only reduces the incidence of non-healing wounds but also results in a relative increase in below knee as opposed to above knee operations. The methods currently available include thermography [16], radioisotope clearance studies [17], photoplethysmography [18], transcutaneous oxygen measurements (TcPO$_2$) [19, 20] and laser Doppler flowmetry [20]. In the future magnetic resonance spectroscopy (MRS) might also be helpful in quantifying the degree of ischaemia at different levels in the limb [21]. Since the determinants of wound healing are multifactorial, it is not reasonable to expect any single objective test to be 100 per cent reliable and clinical judgement must still be exercised, particularly when the results fall within a borderline range. However, it has been pointed out that there is a considerable discrepancy in many centres between detailed investigation of patients being considered for vascular reconstruction and the lack of objective assessment in those who require amputation. Given the technology which is now available and its proven efficacy, the continuation of such practices is difficult to justify.

Opinion is divided about the place of through-knee or Gritti-Stokes amputation. Both are associated with problems of limb fitting because an artificial limb cannot be placed at the same level as the natural knee joint of the contralateral limb. Both procedures are certainly inferior to a below knee amputation but may be preferred to above knee amputations in selected patients, particularly when objective tests indicate borderline skin perfusion at the below knee level [17]. In the United Kingdom these amputations account for less than 3 per cent of the total.

Recommendation 26 of the European Consensus Document states that "Amputations should be followed by appropriate rehabilitation". Ideally there should be consultation between the surgeon, the physiotherapists and the prosthetist at all stages once the need for an amputation has been determined and there should also be facilities for early rehabilitation and limb fitting on site. Unfortunately these ideals cannot always be attained, but the surgeon has prime responsibility to ensure that his patient receives adequate rehabilitation following operation. Proposals that all amputations should be carried out in special limb surgery centres are not practical for the majority of patients at present, nor is it necessarily desirable to transfer a patient with chronic vascular disease to another unit for this one procedure. R 26

Finally it is a common-sense observation that patients should only be subjected to amputation provided that there is a reasonable expectation that he or she will survive the operation and for some time afterwards. In some very elderly and seriously debilitated patients, critical ischaemia may be regarded as a terminal event and palliative treatment with pain relief and nursing care is the preferred option in these circumstances.

## 7.7 Summary

- Primary amputation should only be undertaken if the possibility of revascularisation procedures has been excluded.
- Angiography should always be performed before major amputation in patients with potentially reversible critical ischaemia.
- Prosthetic grafts to the ankle rarely succeed. However, they might still be indicated as an alternative to amputation.
- In some cases primary amputation may be better than subjecting the patient to repeated surgical procedures with little chance of success and increasing mortality and morbidity.
- Below knee amputation is preferred to above knee because of lower morbidity and mortality rates and better mobility following operation.
- Objective measurements of skin perfusion should be employed to aid the selection of the level of amputation wherever possible.
- Amputations should be followed by appropriate rehabilitation.

## References


1. Amputation statistics for England, Wales and Northern Ireland (1986) Department of Health and Social Security, London
2. Harris PL, Read F, Eardley A, Charlesworth D, Wakefield J, Sellwood RA (1974) The fate of elderly amputees. Br J Surg 61:665–668
3. Kannel WB, Skinner JJ, Schwartz MJ, Shurtleff D (1970) Intermittent claudiation – Incidence in the Framingham Study. Circulation XLI, p 875
4. Widmer LK, Biland L, Dasilva A (1985) Risk profile and occlusive peripheral arterial disease (OPAD). In: Proceedings of the 13th International Congress of Angiology
5. Wolfe JHN (1986) Defining the outcome of critical ischaemia: a one year prospective study. Br J Surg 73:321
6. Scarpato R, Gembarowicz R, Forber R et al. (1981) Intraoperative pre-reconstruction arteriography. Arch Surg 116:1953–1955
7. Harris PL, Campbell H (1983) Adjuvant distal arteriovenous shunt with femoro-tibial bypass for critical ischaemia. Br J Surg 70:377–380
8. Beard JD, Scott DJ, Evans JM, Skidmore R, Horrocks M (1988) Pulse generated run-off, a new method of determining calf vessel patency. Br J Surg 74(4):361–363
9. Simms MH (1988) Is pedal arch patency a pre-requisite for successful reconstruction? In: Greenhalgh RM, Jamieson CW, Nicolaides AN (eds) Limb salvage and amputation for vascular disease. Publ Saunders, London, pp 49–62
10. Parvin SD, Evans DH, Bell PRF (1985) Peripheral resistance measurement in the assessment of severe peripheral vascular disease. Br J Surg 72:751–753
11. Ascer E, Veith FH, White-Flores SA et al. (1987) Intraoperative outflow resistance as a predictor of late patency of femoro-popliteal and infra-popliteal arterial bypasses. J Vasc Surg 5:820–827

12. Harris PL, Campbell H (1986) Femoro-distal bypass for critical ischaemia: is the use of prosthetic grafts justified? Ann Vasc Surg 1:66–72
13. Dormandy JA, Thomas PRS (1988) What is the natural history of a critically ischaemic patient with and without his leg? In: Greenhalgh RM, Jamieson CW, Nicolaides AN (eds) Limb salvage and amputation for vascular disease. Publ Saunders, pp 11–26
14. Robinson KP et al. (1982) Skewflap myoplastic below knee amputation. Br J Surg 69(9)
15. Ruckley CV, Prescott RJ (1988) Is there any advantage of skewflap rather than Burgess below knee amputation? In: Greenhalgh RM, Jamieson CW, Nicolaides AN (eds) Limb salvage and amputation for vascular disease. Publ Saunders
16. Spence VA, Walker WF, Troup IM, Murdoch G (1981) Amputation of the ischaemic limb: selection of the optimum site by thermography. Angiology 32:155–169
17. Holstein P (1985) Skin perfusion pressure measured by radioisotope washout for predicting wound healing in lower limb amputation for arterial occlusive disease. Thesis Acta Orthop Scand Suppl 213
18. Stockel M, Oresen J, Bröchner-Mortensen J, Emnius H (1982) Standardised photoelectric technique as routine method for selection of amputation level. Acta Orthop Scand 53:875
19. Ratcliff DA, Clyne CAC, Chant ADB, Webster JHH (1984) Prediction of amputation wound healing: the role of transcutaneous oxygen tension in the selection of amputation level. Am J Surg 147:510–517
20. Fairs SLE, Ham RO, Conway BA, Roberts VC (1987) Limb perfusion in the lower limb amputee – a comparative study using laser Doppler flowmeter and a transcutaneous oxygen electrode. Prosthet Orthot Int 11:80–84
21. Hands LJ, Bore PJ, Galloway G, Morris PJ, Radda GK (1986) Muscle metabolism in patients with peripheral vascular disease investigated by $^{31}$P. NMR spectroscopy. Clin Sci 71:283–290

# *Commentary*

*Felix Mahler and Peter Stirnemann*

We broadly agree with the clear considerations of Harris and Moody and their conclusions that primary amputation should only be undertaken when every possibility of revascularization has been excluded or exhausted. From the experience of our combined medical-surgical team approach to vascular disease, we would like to make a few remarks on non-surgical possibilities in patients who are candidates for amputation and on some aspects concerning amputation level.

Revascularization may consist of reconstructive surgery, catheter revascularization or of a combination of the two. There are reports of surgical limb salvage of 83% [1] or even 97% [2] in the short term, and of about 70% after two years for femoro-distal reconstruction [3]. It is hard to improve on these excellent results using other techniques. Our own analysis from femoro-distal saphenous vein bypasses showed that failures occurred only in those patients with a run-off less than 50 ml per minute [4]. However, even in this poor risk group 82% ended up with a patent bypass, and in only 10% was a major amputation required. However, percutaneous transluminal angioplasty (PTA) also has a place in the treatment of chronic critical limb ischaemia. In the series by Schneider [5] the amputation rate was 23%, and in Zeitler's series [6] 15%. Our own experience [7, 8] of PTA in endangered limbs showed an 18% amputation rate within 6 to 24 months. In situations where PTA is technically appropriate it may be preferable to surgery because of its lesser cost and greater safety.

The question arises whether in cases where reconstruction is not possible, primary or secondary amputation could be avoided by some medical or physical treatment. Many possibilities have been proposed such as intravenous or intra-arterial infusions of vasoactive drugs, as well as alternative methods such as spinal cord stimulation [9], hyperbaric oxygen therapy, etc. Recently most of the discussion has been directed to the prostaglandins $PGE_1$ and $PGI_2$ and its analogues. Naturally these patients represent the poorest selection because they had been considered for revascularization but rejected for a variety of reasons such as poor run-off, high risk of anaesthesia or lack of autologous graft material. Few of the controlled studies with such patients report on amputation rate. Böhme et al. [10] describe a late amputation rate of 34% in a group of patients treated with ATP and of 10% of those treated with $PGE_1$ intra-arterially. Gruss [11] could reduce the rate of minor amputations of 18% in a control group to 2% in a group treated by intra-arterial infusion of $PGE_1$ afterfemoro-distal bypass surgery, but the rate of major amputations was 2% in both groups. In an open study Heidrich [12] reports on an overall amputation rate of about 20% in 202 patients after $PGE_1$ treatment in whom an amputation rate of about 50% was expected. The stable prostacycline analogue iloprost has the advantage of being suitable for intravenous application [13]. With this substance only few controlled studies are available on amputation rates. While ulcer healing seems to be significantly more frequent in the study by Diehm [14] with

55% in the iloprost group and 24% in the placebo group, the amputation rate remained equal in both groups after one year. A few comparable controlled studies exist and some are under way on other drugs such as naftidrofuryl, buflomedil or pentoxyfyllin, but in no case have the results exceeded those with the prostanoids. Uncontrolled studies have to be regarded with reservation because the spontaneous course of the disease is not known even in carefully selected patients.

In conclusion at the moment medical treatment does not present a viable alternative to revascularization. Not only do the drugs lack the high success rate of surgery but they have some disadvantages. They are applied parenterally and usually during several weeks, and they are not free of side effects. However, when revascularization is not possible or has failed, and it the patient does not present with major necrosis, and is able to endure several weeks of medical treatment, a trial with drugs seems to be worthwhile. According to the above results it is clear that the number of patients profiting from this treatment cannot be very high. At present it is not possible to draw definite conclusions, and therefore a careful risk-benefit evaluation has to be done in the case of each patient.

In some cases amputation may remain unavoidable, and, whenever possible, it should be performed at the below-knee level. Amputation at the transgenicular level merits special comment as alternative to the above-knee amputation. In our experience mortality (7% and 8%, respectively) and primary healing rate (44% and 41%, respectively) were comparable in 330 below-knee amputations and in 141 transgenicular amputations [15]. Even though full rehabilitation with 85% was superior in the below-knee amputation than that of 66% in the transgenicular one, they both far exceed that of 25% in the above-knee amputee. This supports the view that the transgenicular level is preferable to the above-knee amputation whenever rehabilitation of the patient is envisaged.

### *References*


1. LoGerfo FW, Corson JD, Mannick JA (1977) Improved results with femoropopliteal vein grafts for limb salvage. Arch Surg 112:567
2. Reichle Fa, Martinson MW, Rankin KP (1980) Infrapopliteal arterial reconstruction in the severly ischemic lower extremity. Ann Surg 191:59–65
3. Largiader J (1987) Gefäßchirurgie am Unterschenkel. Huber, Bern
4. Stirnemann P, Triller J (1986) The fate of femoropopliteal and femorodistal bypass grafts in relation to intraoperative flow measurement: an analysis of 100 consecutive reconstructions for limb salvage. Surgery 100:38–44
5. Schneider E, Grüntzig A, Bollinger A (1983) PTA for limb salvage – progress in therapy for severe leg ischemia with rest pain and gangrene. In: Dotter CT, Grüntzig A, Schoop W, Zeitler E (eds) Percutaneous Transluminal Angioplasty. Springer, Berlin Heidelberg New York, pp 222–226
6. Zeitler E, Richter E, Roth F, Schoop W (1982) Results of percutaneous transluminal angioplasty. Radiology 146:57–60
7. Gallino A, Mahler F, Probst P, Nachbur B (1984) Percutaneous transluminal angioplasty of the arteries of the lower limbs: a 5 year follow-up. Circulation 70:619–623
8. Mahler F (1990) Katheterinterventionen in der Angiologie. Thieme, Stuttgart
9. Jacobs MJHM, Jörning PJG, Joshi SR, Kitslaar PJEHM, Slaaf DW, Reneman RS (1988) Epidural spinal cord electrical stimulation improves microvascular blood flow in severe limb ischemia. Ann Surg 207:179–183

10. Böhme H, Brülisauer M, Härtel U, Bollinger A (1988) Kontrollierte Zweizentren-Studie zur Wirksamkeit von intraarteriellen Prostaglandin E1-Infusionen bei peripherer arterieller Verschlußkrankheit im Stadium II and IV.In: Heidrich H, Böhme H, Rogatti W (eds) Prostaglandin E1 Wirkungen und therapeutische Wirksamkeit. Springer, Berlin Heidelberg New York, pp 118–123
11. Gruss JD, Fietze-Fischer B (1988) Die adjuvante PGE1 Therapie bei femoro-distalen Rekonstruktionen. In: Heidrich H, Böhme H, Rogatti W (eds) Prostaglandin E1 Wirkungen und therapeutische Wirksamkeit. Springer, Berlin Heidelberg New York, pp 151–180
12. Heidrich H, Ranft J, Peters A, Rummel S (1988) Intravenöse Prostavasin-Therapie bei peripherarteriellen Durchblutungsstörungen im Fontaine-Stadium III und IV. Früh- und Spätergebnisse einer Screening-Studie. In: Heidrich H, Böhme H, Rogatti W (eds) Prostaglandin E1 Wirkungen und therapeutische Wirksamkeit. Springer, Berlin Heidelberg New York, pp 112–117
13. Oberender H, Krais Th, Schäfer M, Belcher G (1989) Clinical benefits of iloprost, a stable prostacyclin (PGI2) analog, in severe peripheral arterial disease (PAD). Advances in Prostaglandin, Thromboxane, and Leukotriene Research 19:311–316
14. Diehm C, Abri O, Baitsch G, Bechara G, Beck K, Breddin HK, Brock FE, Clevert HD, Corovic D, Marshall M, Rahmel B, Scheffler P, Schmidt W, Oberender HA (1989) Iloprost, ein stabiles Prostacyclinderivat, bei arterieller Verschlußkrankheit im Stadium IV. Dtsch Med Wochenschr 114:783–788
15. Stirnemann P, Mlinaric Z, Oesch A, Kirchhof B, Althaus U (1987) Major lower extremity amputation in patients with peripheral arterial insufficiency with special reference to the transgenicular amputation. J Cardiovasc Surg 28:152–158

# Chapter 8

## Primary Pharmacotherapy other than Prostanoids

Marc Verstraete and Raymond Verhaeghe



The high morbidity and mortality from critical limb ischaemia as well as from less severe derangement of the arterial blood supply in the legs, has promoted the continuing search for effective methods for its prevention and treatment. Although in most instances atherosclerosis of medium sized arteries and also of smaller arteries in diabetes, is the underlying disorder leading to critical limb ischaemia, platelet aggregation and fibrin deposition on atheromatous lesions may further reduce blood flow (see Chapter 3). Drugs interfering with the activation of platelets (antiplatelet drugs, prostanoids) and coagulation factors (heparin and oral anticoagulants, hirudin, defibrinogenating agents, thrombolytic drugs) will therefore be considered in this overview. The clinical usefulness of hyperbaric oxygen, plasma expanders and vasoactive drugs are also briefly discussed.

## 8.1 Pharmacology of Drugs Under Consideration

### 8.1.1 Antiplatelet Agents

There is convincing evidence that platelets play a central role in the formation of a thrombus on an atherosclerotic vessel wall; it is even possible that platelets contribute to the development of the atherosclerotic lesions themselves. Considering that the formation of a platelet thrombus may be seen as the uncontrolled expansion of the physiological function of platelets, it is appropriate to briefly describe how platelets are activated in order to better understand how this process can be inhibited with antiplatelet drugs (see Section 3.3.3).

In normal conditions platelets are quiescent and circulate freely in the blood as they do not adhere on the normal vascular endothelium. When the endothelium lining is lost at the site of vessel injury or at the level of a ruptured atherosclerotic plaque, the exposed subendothelial tissue provides a surface to which platelets can adhere. Among the constituents of normal subendothelium, the various types of collagen and its ubiquitous companion, fibronectin, are readily interacting with platelets, more particulary with glycoproteins (e.g. Ia) located on their membrane. This initial bond is strengthened by the interaction of several adhesive proteins. One of them is a large multimeric plasma protein termed von Willebrand factor capable of binding not only to exposed subendothelial collagen but also to the platelet membrane glycoproteins Ib and IIb/IIIa. This macromolecule thereby stabilizes the attachment of platelets to the vessel wall. The platelets constituting this monolayer soon become activated and release mediators, like adenosine diphosphate (ADP) and thromboxane $A_2$ capable of recruiting additional circulating platelets which bind to and transform the initial monolayer into a platelet aggregate. In this activation process, the conformation of the platelet membrane glycoprotein IIb/IIIa complex changes, so that it can interact with plasma fibrinogen (via a unique dodecapeptide sequence in its gamma chain as well as via a second tripeptide sequence on its alpha chain) and with other adhesive proteins (fibronectin, thrombospondin). Fibrinogen thus serves to link platelets together into a tighter aggregate. These processes in platelets are associated with complex signal transductions, regulated by specific agonists (ADP, thrombin, epinephrine, serotonin, thromboxane $A_2$, PAF, ...) that bind to specific platelet receptors and activate the hydrolysis of phosphatidylinositol. The resulting products of hydrolysis can then induce a transient increase in intracellular calcium and activate an intracellular protein kinase that phosphorylates intraplatelet regulatory proteins. Finally, the eicosanoids derived from arachidonic acid in platelets, leukocytes, and endothelial cells provide short-acting biological mediators further promoting platelet activation and local vasoconstriction. Aggregated platelets provide a surface on which coagulation factors can concentrate, making their interaction much more likely than in the fluid phase of the blood.

Aspirin inactivates cyclooxygenase in platelets and endothelial cells, a key enzyme in prostaglandin synthesis. Platelets, in contrast to endothelial cells, are unable to replenish cyclooxygenase during their lifespan and thus the formation of the vasoconstricting and platelet aggregating thromboxane $A_2$ is blocked. Higher doses are required to inhibit cyclooxygenase in endothelial cells than in platelets. A daily dose of 50 mg of aspirin inhibits 80–98% of platelet thromboxane $A_2$-production and changes platelet function and bleeding time to the same extent as a 10-fold excess dose of the drug. Low-dose aspirin has but trivial effects on vascular, gastric and renal cyclooxygenase activity.

Ticlopidine is a thienopyridine that inhibits ADP-induced aggregation and prolongs the bleeding time; it probably modifies the ADP-receptor in platelets and inhibits the fibrinogen binding to the glycoprotein IIb–IIIa on the platelet membrane.

A more recent approach in this field is the development of specific thromboxane synthetase inhibitors. These substances inhibit thromboxane formation and reorientate cyclic endoperoxide towards other prostaglandins such as prostaglandin $D_2$ and eventually prostacyclin. They do, however, not inhibit the formation of proaggregatory cyclic endoperoxides and their net action is therefore again subject to a complex balance of pro- and antiaggregating prostaglandins. A next step forward is the development of specific and safe thromboxane/cyclic endoperoxide receptor antagonists followed by drugs which combine the characteristics of the two classes of agents [1, 2]. The potential usefulness of these new approaches has to be verified in clinical trials.

### 8.1.2 Heparin

Heparin, a mucopolysaccharide extracted from bovine lung tissue and intestinal mucosa of pigs and cattle, is a natural anticoagulant, the activity of which is related to its strong electronegative charge, forming complexes with positively charged proteins.

By attaching itself to the lysine-binding sites of antithrombin III, heparin induces a conformational change in this protein and allows the reactive site arginine to reach and thereby to inhibit the active serine site of thrombin, activated factor X (factor Xa) and also of other serine proteases (the activated forms of factors IX, XI, XII, kallikrein and plasmin). At least 16 to 20 monosaccharide units per heparin molecule (circa 4800 daltons) are necessary for full expression of the potential ability of antithrombin to inhibit thrombin. The binding of thrombin to heparin is of an electrostatic nature and strongly depends on the length of the heparin molecule: the greater the molecule, the greater is the ability of thrombin to diffuse along the heparin chain into the antithrombin III molecule which is also bound to heparin. In this "sliding" model, an increase in chain length of heparin results in an increased reaction rate because of a higher probability of interaction between thrombin and heparin in solution.

The inhibition of factor Xa is due to the formation of a binary complex between antithrombin III and factor Xa, in which heparin binds and activates antithrombin III but does not bind Xa. Low molecular weight heparin molecules result in factor Xa inactivation, provided they contain the antithrombin III binding domain, but may be too small to form a complex with antithrombin III and thrombin. Small heparin fractions will thus selectively inhibit factor Xa.

Heparin binds reversibly to its target sites of action. About two-thirds of the mass of heparin, which is associated with around 15% of its anticoagulant activity, has a low binding affinity for antithrombin III, while the remaining third, which is associated with 85% of its anticoagulant activity, has a high affinity for antithrombin III. The region where high affinity heparin binds to antithrombin III has been defined by characterisation of oligosaccharides. Only a limited number of heparin molecules contain the required saccharide sequence. Moreover, histidine-rich glycoprotein competes with antithrombin III for binding of heparin, thereby neutralising its anticoagulant activity. Complex formation with a third heparin-dependent inhibitor, termed cofactor II, predominates at high heparin concentrations (over 5 units/ml plasma). Heparin has a short plasma half-life of 1 to 2 hours which varies widely between individuals.

The disappearance of the anticoagulant activity of heparin follows non linear kinetics and is compatible with a model based on the combination of a saturable mechanism (most probably rapid uptake by the endothelium and desulphation by mononuclear phagocytes) and a linear mechanism (most probably elimination by the kidney). The faster disappearance of the thrombin inhibitor activity (anti-IIa activity) than the anti-factor Xa activity in the initial clearance phase also suggests an earlier elimination mechanism of large molecules having a high anti-IIa/anti-Xa ratio.

### 8.1.3 Oral Anticoagulants

The oral anticoagulants are synthetic compounds of two chemical types – coumarin and indanedione derivatives. Both types act by inhibiting the synthesis of biologically active prothrombin, factors VII, IX and X, and proteins C and S. The normal synthesis of these six coagulation factors requires vitamin K. Oral anticoagulants inhibit the normal action of vitamin K, resulting in the accumulation of biologically inactive derivatives of clotting factors. These derivatives may represent a common precursor or incomplete individual coagulation factors. Active clotting factors are formed by carboxylation of their precursor proteins during which vitamin K-hydroquinone is oxidised to a vitamin K epoxide. Oral anticoagulants prevent the reduction of this biologically inactive epoxide back into active vitamin K-hydroquinone by blocking an intrahepatic epoxide reductase. This, in turn, prevents the formation of di-gamma carboxylglutamic acid (Gla) residues on the six coagulation proteins mentioned above, thereby reducing their activity.

Oral anticoagulants are therefore indirect inactivating drugs and all require a delay before their action is seen. The delay of their effects depends on the clearance (half-life) from the circulation of the coagulation factors, the final synthesis of which is inhibited, and on the extent of this inhibition, which in turn depends on the induction dose. Factor VII, which has the shortest half-life, decreases first, followed by factors IX and X, protein C and S, and prothrombin. Although coumarin therapy decreases the activity of certain coagulants and anticoagulants, the net effect is to impair coagulation and reduce the rate of thrombus formation.

### 8.1.4 Hirudin

Hirudin is a natural polypeptide with very specific antithrombin activity, isolated from the salivary glands of the leech *Hirudo medicinalis*. The protein was isolated and characterized [3]. Natural hirudin is a potent and specific inhibitor of human thrombin ($Ki = 2 \times 10^{-12}$) forming an inactive equimolar complex. The formed complex is very stable under normal physiological conditions. All catalytic functions of complexed thrombin are blocked. The major recognition areas seem to be located between position 40 and 48 of the hirudin amino sequence which contains the cleavage site for thrombin. The hirudin-thrombin complex can be dissociated by acidification or heating, whereby thrombin is denatured and hirudin released in its active form.

The gene for hirudin has been synthesized, cloned and expressed in yeast by recombinant DNA technology [4]. The kinetic constants (inhibition of thrombin) of recombinant hirudin are similar to that observed with natural hirudin [5]. Also the pharmacokinetics in laboratory animals and man of natural and recombinant hirudin are very similar and can best be described by an open two-compartment model with first order kinetics, thus a constant fraction of drug present is eliminated per unit of time. After intravenous administration, hirudin plasma levels decline biphasically with half-lives of 10–15 min and 50–100 min for distribution and elimination phase, respectively.

### 8.1.5 Thrombolytic Agents

These agents include: (a) proteolytic enzymes acting directly on fibrin, e.g. plasmin, trypsin and Aspergillus proteases (brinase), and (b) drugs capable of activating plasminogen, either directly e.g. pro-urokinase (saruplase), urokinase and tissue-type plasminogen activator (t-PA or alteplase), or indirectly (e.g. streptokinase and anisoylated streptokinase human plasminogen complex or anistreplase). The plasminogen activators are serine proteases with a high specificity for plasminogen, which hydrolyse the Arg560-Val561 peptide bond, yielding the active plasmin.

Streptokinase is a nonenzyme protein, a catalytic by-product of group beta-haemolytic streptococci; its molecular weight is 47000. Streptokinase forms a 1:1 stoichiometric complex with plasminogen which then undergoes a transition exposing an active site in the modified plasminogen moiety, whereby the complex becomes a potent plasminogen activator. Highly purified preparations are commercially available and are usually well tolerated. Therapeutic plasma concentrations are rapidly achieved and can be sustained for several days, if necessary. The antigenicity of streptokinase in man is a disadvantage and prevents retreatment within the first 3 months of a previous course, as a consequence of a sustained rise of antistreptokinase antibodies induced during treatment.

Anisoylated streptokinase-human plasminogen activator complex is an inactive derivative obtained by acylation of the active site serine (APSAC, anistreplase). It reactivates at physiological pH following spontaneous deacylation.

Urokinase is a trypsin-like enzyme composed of two polypeptide chains connected by a disulfide bridge, which activates plasminogen directly to plasmin. This naturally occurring plasminogen activator is excreted in human urine, from which it can be extracted; urokinase may also be isolated from tissue cultures of human embryonic kidney cells. Purified urokinase preparations are nonantigenic, non-pyrogenic and their proper use is most often associated with a milder coagulation defect than that with streptokinase, but with a similar incidence of bleeding to that shown for streptokinase treated patients.

Single-chain urokinase-type plasminogen activator (scu-PA, saruplase) or pro-urokinase is a single-chain glycoprotein containing 411 amino acids, which is converted to urokinase by hydrolysis of the Lys158-Ile159 peptide bond. Saruplase has very little activity towards low molecular weight substrates but has intrinsic plasminogen-activating potential, however, with a catalytic efficacy that is two orders of magnitude lower than that of urokinase.

Tissue-type plasminogen activator (t-PA or alteplase) is a trypsin like serine protease composed of 527 amino acids which occurs either as a single-chain glycoprotein or as a two-chain proteolytic derivative. Alteplase is a poor plasminogen activator in the absence of fibrin, but it binds specifically to fibrin and activates plasminogen at the fibrin surface several hundred-fold more efficiently than in the circulation.

### 8.1.6 Defibrinogenating Agents

Defibrinogenation is a form of haemorheology that aims at enhancing blood flow by enzymatically lowering plasma fibrinogen and thus decreasing plasma viscosity and red cell aggregation.

The defibrinogenating agents currently available are enzymes derived from snake venom – ancrod from the venom of the Malayan swamp viper *Agkistrodon rhodostoma* Boie and batroxobin from the *Bothrops moojeni* and *Bothrops marajoensis* snakes. Both agents remove only one peptide (fibrinopeptide A) from fibrinogen and the resulting monomers are polymerised into atypical fibrin. As they do not activate factor XIII which normally cross links the fibrin, the unstable fibrin "microclots" are probably removed by activation of the endogenous fibrinolytic enzyme system and through phagocytosis by the reticuloendothelial system. Since the two agents affect only fibrinogen, the entire anticoagulant effect is therefore due to the resulting fibrinogen depletion and their effect is easy to measure. Provided they are administered slowly, intravascular fibrin can be cleared as it is formed and the effect is termed therapeutic defibrinogenation [6, 7]. Ancrod and batroxobin are foreign proteins and induce formation of antibodies which can neutralise their effect. This can be overcome by increasing the dose when the antibodies appear, but this is only effective for 2 or 3 weeks, after which time treatment becomes ineffective. Antibodies disappear within 6 months and prevent retreatment before this time.

### 8.1.7 Drugs for Normovolaemic Haemodilution

Dextran is a colloid, composed of glucose molecules. These chains are formed by an enzymatic action of the bacteria *Leuconostoc mesenteroides* on sucrose. The molecular weight of these molecules can be several millions, but to be used clinically it should not exceed 100000. A decrease in the molecular weight can be accomplished by fractionation of the molecules. On the other hand the molecular weight should not be lower than about 40000, in order to remain in the circulation for a reasonable length of time.

Dextran is a reliable plasma volume expander comparable to albumin, and definitely superior to homologous plasma. Dextran is now available as a 10% solution with a mean molecular weight of 40000, and a 6% solution with a mean molecular weight of 70000. The plasma volume expanding effect of the latter lasts slightly longer than the former preparation but has, however, the advantage of really decreasing the blood viscosity, even at an unchanged haematocrit. It is of importance to stress that all dextran is completely eliminated from the circulation within a few days, partly by elimination via the urine, partly by metabolism.

It was demonstrated that dextran 40 also has flow improving capacities. This is partly effected by a simple decrease in haematocrit, which is a factor of decisive influence on the blood viscosity. Furthermore dextran 40 has an effect to decrease the blood viscosity even when the haematocrit is unchanged. Dextran of low molecular weight also counteracts the red cell aggregation.

A third property of dextran is its antithrombotic effect. Dextran coats both platelets and vascular endothelial cells and increases their electronegativity; it also produces a decrease in factor VIII-related antigen, out of proportion to what could be expected by dilution effects alone. Both combine to produce a situation similar to that seen in von Willebrand's disease. Dextran also facilitates plasminogen activation and inhibits alpha 2-antiplasmin and plasminogen activator inhibitor, thereby accelerating plasma clot lysis. Fibrin polymerized in the presence of dextran is structurally modified and is more easily lysed and less platelet reactive.

Hydroxyethyl starch (HES) is another plasma expander with unexplained rheological properties. It inhibits platelet aggregation and high concentrations may also inhibit red cell aggregation. Elimination of HES from the body can be delayed in patients with impaired renal function, leading to a risk of hypervolaemia.

### 8.1.8 Hyperbaric Oxygen

Oxygen is carried in the blood both chemically, combined with haemoglobin and physically dissolved in plasma, only the former being important under normal circumstances. At normal oxygen pressure, one litre of blood contains about 200 ml (20 vol%) of oxygen as oxyhaemoglobin and 3 ml (0.3 vol%) in solution in the plasma. The degree to which a gas enters into physical solution in fluids is in direct proportion to the partial pressure of the gas to which the fluid is exposed (Henry's law) and consequently when the tension of the inspired oxygen is raised the oxygen content of the plasma also rises. By increasing the pressure to three atmospheres absolute (ata) the amount of physically dissolved oxygen in the capillaries should rise to 6.6 vol%, a 22-fold increase.

The oxygen requirements of the tissue can therefore be met by the oxygen dissolved physically in the plasma. This fraction diffuses freely in the interstitial fluid.

Hyperbaric oxygen inhalation provokes two types of vasomotor reactions. Vasoconstriction occurs in normally oxygenated tissues: autoregulation leads to a proportional decrease of the arterial inflow to avoid high tissue oxygen tension when the arterial oxygen supply increases. At the same time vasodilatation occurs in ischaemic areas: an increased flow to ischaemic limbs can be demonstrated by plethysmography and should lead to a massive supply of hyperoxygenated blood to hypoxic tissue.

### 8.1.9 Vasoactive Drugs

More than a dozen different drugs are recommended for the treatment of patients with arterial insufficiency of the limb or cerebral circulation and any newcomer is claimed to be superior to the previous compounds. This suggests that pharmacological treatment is less than satisfactory. There is no doubt that many of these compounds have been shown to increase blood flow to the limbs in normal animals; some also do so in healthy man. Whether the same agents can increase the blood supply in hypoxaemic areas of patients with occlusive vascular disease is often uncertain; such an effect has been demonstrated only for a very few agents.

Admittedly, the clinical pharmacology and critical clinical evaluation of these substances is very difficult, as is the transposition of their pharmacological effects from healthy man to patients with obliterative arterial disorders. Muscle flow at rest is usually normal in these patients and dilating the vessels located distally to the arterial obstruction may not increase blood flow if the resistance of the collateral vessels remains fixed. During exercise, the pressure beyond the main obstruction may even become lower; the tension of the contracting muscle can exceed this reduced pressure and hence impede blood flow. Furthermore, the clinical effects of ischaemia in the limbs are manifest in two physiologically different vascular areas, namely skin and muscle. $\beta$-Adrenoceptor agonists may increase muscle flow, but have little effect on skin flow where predominantly $\alpha$-receptors are present. Conversely, sympathetic nervous system blocking agents would primarily affect skin vessels since there is little vasoconstrictor tone in skeletal muscle. It is therefore conceivable that a given "vasodilator" compound would not be useful in every clinical condition in this field; discriminate, specific recommendations should therefore be supported by separate clinical trials.

To be useful, an anticlaudication agent should act on the blood flow of the hypoxaemic muscles only. If it does not possess selectivity, it may dilate much more readily normal arteries in the healthier limbs than the obliterated arteries of the limping leg. Not only will this diversion of blood flow further deprive the ischaemic leg with its higher resistance, but a reduction in the systemic pressure may also result, more particularly at exercise, due to additional vasodilatation in active muscles. The resulting decrease in the head of pressure may critically affect the perfusion pressure in the most ischaemic leg. Very few clinical reports with experimental agents mention repeated systemic and local pressure measurements during exercise both in the ischaemic and less affected leg.

## 8.2 Clinical Use

### 8.2.1 Antiplatelet Agents

To date, aspirin and ticlopidine are the only two antiplatelet drugs which have been shown to retard the progression of atherosclerosis and the occurrence of its thrombotic complications in legs of patients with obstructive arterial disease. Three hundred patients with a stenosis of the femoral artery were randomized by Schoop et al. [8] to receive daily either 1 g of aspirin, 1 g of aspirin combined with 225 mg of dipyridamole or placebo; they were followed up to 4 years. The occlusion rate was lower in the two groups treated with the active drugs, but the combination was not superior to the administration of aspirin alone. In addition, antiplatelet therapy did not prevent femoral artery thrombosis in diabetic and hypertensive patients. Hess et al. [9] reported a placebo-controlled, double-blind, 2 year trial in 199 patients with arteriographically studied evolution of peripheral atherosclerosis. Plaque progression rate was most pronounced in the placebo group, less so in the aspirin-treated group (1 g daily) and least of all in the aspirin-dipyridamole-treated group (1 g, 225 mg daily). In contrast with the results of Schoop et al. [8], patients who continued to smoke and those with hypertension benefited most from active treatment (see also Section 3.3.3). In a placebo-controlled randomized trial in 114 claudicants ticlopidine significantly reduced progression of the disease as shown by arteriograms repeated one year later [10]. Ticlopidine inhibits the binding of fibrinogen to its receptor on platelets, the glycoprotein IIb/IIIa and possibly modifies the ADP receptor [11]. All these trials did not specifically select patients with critical ischaemia. In addition, they did not study clinical endpoints. In a Japanese trial [12] ticlopidine appeared to significantly decrease the number and extent of ischaemic ulcers due to atherosclerosis and thromboangiitis obliterans. The effect of other antiplatelet drugs in the treatment of critical leg ischaemia has not been investigated.

Patients with peripheral occlusive arterial disease have a poor general prognosis with an excess cardiovascular mortality and morbidity. Whether antiplatelet drugs favourably influence this poor outcome in patients with peripheral atherosclerosis as they appear to do to some extent in patients after a first coronary or cerebrovascular event, has thus far not been investigated. The antiserotonin agent ketanserin did not reduce the cardiovascular mortality, nor the incidence of non-fatal vascular events in a large multicentre trial with almost 4000 claudication patients [13].

### 8.2.2 Unfractionated and Low Molecular Weight Heparin

No clinical trials have been published on the use of unfractionated heparin for treatment of patients with rest pain and ulcers. In an open trial, Fraciparin (CY 216), a low molecular weight heparin fraction, was administered subcutaneously in 40 patients with leg ulcers mainly due to atherosclerosis, including diabetic patients. A decrease of rest pain and healing of ulcers previously resistant to treatment was noted [14]. These preliminary results were encouraging enough to organize an ongoing comparative randomised clinical trial.

### 8.2.3 Oral Anticoagulants

Thrombosis of atherosclerotic arteries is only the final step of a long evolution of the underlying disorder. Therefore, long-term oral anticoagulation is unlikely to represent a spectacular advance in the prevention of progression of peripheral arterial occlusive disease. In fact, a few trials have shown a favourable trend with oral anticoagulants, but their design and size do not allow a definite conclusion (reviewed by Bounameaux et al. [15]). A prospective study [16] was performed in patients suffering from intermittent claudication. All the selected patients were initially on oral anticoagulant therapy for at least 6 months. They were then randomly assigned to switch to placebo or to continue oral anticoagulation. The trial was stopped prematurely because of a significant greater number of deaths in the placebo group. These favourable results were apparently not confirmed in a second placebo controlled but still unpublished trial [17], which showed no benefit of anticoagulants on total mortality, although the progression of the vascular disease (peripheral, cerebrovascular, cardiovascular) appeared delayed.

To examine whether oral anticoagulants given after autologous saphenous bypass surgery at the femoro-popliteal level influenced patient survival, 199 patients were recruited for a controlled randomized clinical trial [18]. The median survival for all patients was at least 60 months. The two groups differed significantly in probability of survival: 10 patients died in the anticoagulant and 20 in the control group. This difference remained significant when patients with an occluded graft (11 in the anticoagulant and 17 in the control group) were excluded from analysis. A large proportion of the patients selected for this trial apparently fulfilled the current definition of critical ischaemia.

### 8.2.4 Hirudin

No clinical trials with hirudin have so far been published.

### 8.2.5 Thrombolytic Agents and Other Proteases

Systemic thrombolytic therapy with streptokinase or urokinase has been used in patients with chronic arterial obstruction, severe ischaemia and poor operative prognosis [19–22] (see also Chapter 5). In the last years, local thrombolysis or the delivery of a thrombolytic agent directly into the thrombus appears to be a more efficient means of achieving rapid clot dissolution, also requiring a lower dose and avoiding to some extent a systemic lytic state. In patients presenting with ischaemia so severe as to threaten the viability of the limb if perfusion is not restored within the next several hours, the most expeditious treatment should be provided. In some patients this may be regional thrombolysis, while in others surgical intervention may be easier and quicker to accomplish. No randomized trial has been performed to determine whether one approach is superior to the other on short or long term [23]. In daily practice, surgery is the first choice in the majority of patients with thrombolysis being reserved for cases in which reconstruction is impractical. In 22 patients with acute limb threatening ischaemia and distal extension of the thrombus, Delcour et al. [24] infused streptokinase intra-arterially and obtained a lytic response in 16 with a complete clinical recovery in 4 only. After a secondary procedure, either angioplasty or surgery, 6 still needed a distal minor amputation.

Local thrombolysis is more commonly used in patients with chronic leg ischaemia. The average success rate in femoro-popliteal occlusion is around 70% and in thrombosis of surgical grafts around 50 to 55% (reviewed by Serradimigni and Villain [25]). In our own experience, the lysis rate is significantly higher in patients with claudication only than in those with advanced stages of ischaemia [26].

Complications of the procedure are haematomas at the arterial puncture site, distal embolization, catheter thrombosis and subintimal dissection. Series in which no distant bleeding is observed are rather rare.

A randomized, single-blind trial of repeated infusions of brinase was carried out in 64 patients with rest pain, necrotic skin defects and/or gangrenous lesions who were candidates for lumbar sympathectomy or amputation [27]. Patients allocated to brinase treatment had a significant increase in calf and ankle pressure indices, indicating that the enzyme was able to augment distal flow in the limb. At six months follow-up, the clinical results were statistically in favour of brinase when all patients were considered, but not if 10 patients with Buerger's disease were omitted from the analysis. Patients treated with a combination of brinase and coumarin had a better clinical outcome than patients receiving either treatment on its own.

A highly purified preparation of hyaluronidase of bovine origin has been used in patients with occlusion of the superficial femoral artery or of branches of the popliteal artery in whom surgical vascular correction was impossible. Hyaluronidase is thought to reduce the size of the ischaemic zone adjacent to the infarcted tissue. It increases capillary permeability and promotes increased diffusion through the extravascular space, reducing oedema and probably assisting in the delivery of oxygen to the ischaemic cells. The encouraging results of an open pilot trial suggested the need to proceed with a clinical trial of intra-arterial hyaluronidase against thymoxamine or prostacyclin [28].

### 8.2.6 Clinical Use of Defibrinogenating Drugs

Although the principle of defibrinogenation is well understood and its effects on haemorheology well demonstrated (lower viscosity and better perfusion), the clinical evaluation of defibrinogenating agents in peripheral ischaemia is far from being straightforward. Early trials, mainly open, reported promising clinical results in 50–80% of the treated patients: relief of pain, reduction in analgesic consumption, better healing of skin ulcers, presumed decrease in amputation frequency and an increase in pain-free walking distance. Some studies even reported objective improvement in flow, distal pressure or muscle $pO_2$. A few controlled but non-blind studies appeared to confirm these promising findings (reviewed by Ernst [29]).

Two placebo-controlled and double-blind trials with ancrod as defibrinogenating agent have been published. Lowe et al. [30] found a remarkable placebo effect in two thirds of 27 patients with critical ischaemia but no significant difference between ancrod and placebo treated patients in analgesic consumption, systolic pressure ratio or number of surgical interventions in the six months following treatment. Although this study has often been criticized for its short treatment period (8 days), at least some effect might have been anticipated if defibrinogenation were at all beneficial. In another trial, 42 patients with critical ischaemia were treated for 3 weeks [31]. Pain was relieved in one quarter of all patients but neither healing of ischaemic ulcers nor subsequent amputation rate were different between verum and placebo. Martin et al. [50] studied the effect of defibrinogenation with batroxobin versus placebo for 21 days in 20 claudication patients and found no difference in walking distance or ankle pressure between the two groups.

Thus, there is no convincing evidence that defibrinogenation is of any clinical value in severe leg ischaemia. The discrepancy in results from open and controlled trials may be due to a strong placebo effect in open studies, although a difference in patient selection is not excluded.

### 8.2.7 Normovolaemic Haemodilution

Normovolaemic haemodilution as a method of treatment for leg ischaemia consists of repeated venesection, combined with infusion of plasma expanders to compensate the volume loss. The aim is to improve leg perfusion by reducing the haematocrit to around 35 or 40%. However, the evidence for a clinical benefit in patients with severe ischaemia is still scarce. Uncontrolled studies show some subjective improvement, eventually substantiated by objective measurements. Very few controlled studies have been conducted. Ernst et al. [32] reported a significant improvement in walking distance and in resting leg flow in stable claudicants treated with haemodilution when compared to placebo. Haemodilution was obtained by weekly venesection and infusion of hydroxy-ethyl starch for 3 weeks. Stolz et al. [33] infused dextran 40 000 in 18 atherosclerotic patients with critical leg ischaemia and skin ulcers. None of them were suitable for reconstructive vascular surgery and 16 had also diabetes. They received daily intravenous infusions of 500 ml dextran and 10 mg deproteinised haemoderivative for 3 to 22 days. Haemodilution resulted in a significant decrease in the rate of above-knee amputation, from 56% to 41% when compared to a historical group of 242 comparable patients (158 diabetics). These results confirm an earlier equally open study of the same group [34].

### 8.2.8 Hyperbaric Oxygen

The initial reports on the use of hyperbaric oxygen in patients with early gangrene of the legs were encouraging as relief of pain was obtained and amputation could be postponed, even for several years [35, 36]. In another study 18 percent of diabetic patients with ulcers refractory to conventional treatment healed completely but all made a fair response. Seventy-five percent of atherosclerotic ulcers in nondiabetic patients improved sufficiently to allow patients to return home and resume daily activities [37]. The longest and largest experience was reported by Fredenucci [38]. He collected more than 2000 patients treated in over 70 000 sessions between 1966 and 1983. Patients with skin ulcers received 1-hour sessions twice daily at a pressure of 2 to 2.5 atm. Relief of rest pain and healing of limiting ulcers was observed in one third of those patients after 4 to 6 weeks of treatment. Not only is the method cumbersome, but it is also unclear to what extent the clinical results can be attributed to concomitant local therapy and heparin infusion.

### 8.2.9 Vasoactive Drugs

Since the case against vasodilating agents was presented [39, 40], new randomized, placebo-controlled, double-blind trials with different agents (pentoxifylline, naftidrofuryl, buflomedil) have been published in claudication patients [41–43]. With these substances, characteristics other than vasodilatation are stressed (for example, improvement in blood rheology or cell oxygenation, vasorecruitment, ...). Atherosclerotic blood vessels are hyperresponsive to serotonin; collateral blood vessels also demonstrate enhanced sensitivity to serotonin. This may have a greater effect on perfusion than the contractile effect of serotonin at the level of the "fixed" atherosclerotic obstruction. Serotonergic blockade with ketanserin inhibits the reduction of collateral blood flow due to an acute thrombosis or to serotonin administration in experimental animal models [44, 45]. Recently, ketanserin was suggested to improve substantially the walking distance and the calf blood flow in patients with claudication [46], but these data have not been confirmed [13, 47].

### 8.2.10 Increase of Systemic Arterial Pressure

Many years ago Lassen et al. [48] reported a successful attempt to treat patients with gangrenous foot ulcers by increasing the systemic arterial pressure with oral sodium chloride supplements (5 to 10 g/24 h) and mineralocortisteroids (see also section 4.2.2). However, increasing the blood pressure in aged atherosclerotic patients is not devoid of risk in terms of cerebral bleeding, and an increase in sodium chloride in the diet may precipitate heart failure. This therapy has been restricted to ischaemic ulcers in young patients with Buerger's disease [49].

## 8.3 Conclusion

Rather few studies on primary pharmacotherapy in arterial obstructive disease deal with patients who suffer from critical leg ischaemia as a separate target group. It is uncertain whether data from patients with less severe ischaemia can be extrapolated to patients with a poorer diagnosis.

This is especially true for antithrombotic drugs, the primary aim of which is to prevent further deterioration. Local thrombolysis requires further testing before a recommendation can be made. The technique may be applicable to certain subgroups of patients: those with a rather short obstruction appear to be the best candidates but surgery is the preferred treatment when applicable. The present results with defibrinogenating agents, haemodilution and vasoactive substances are not convincing or even disappointing.

## References

1. Gresele P, Deckmyn H, Arnout J, Nenci GG, Vermylen J (1989) Characterization of N,N′-bis(3-picolyl)-4-methoxy-isophtalamide (picotamide) as a dual thromboxane $A_2$ receptor antagonist in human platelets. Thromb Haemost 61:479–484
2. Hoet B, Falcon C, De Reys S, Arnout J, Deckmyn H, Vermylen J (1990) R68070, a combined thromboxane/endoperoxide receptor antagonist and thromboxane synthase inhibitor, inhibits human platelet activation in vitro and in vivo: a comparison with aspirin. Blood (in press)

3. Walsmann P, Marckwardt F (1985) On the isolation of the thrombin inhibitor hirudin. Thromb Res 49:563–569
4. Meyhack B, Heim J, Rink H, Zimmermann W, Maerki W (1987) Desulfatohirudin, a specific thrombin inhibitor: expression and secretion in yeast. Thromb Res Suppl 7:33
5. Brown PJ, Dennis S, Hofsteenge J, Stone SR (1988) Use of site directed mutagenesis to investigate the basis for the specificity of Hirudin. Biochemistry 27:6517–6522
6. Bell WR, Pitney WR, Goodwin JF (1968) Therapeutic defibrination in the treatment of thrombotic disease. Lancet 1:490
7. Dormandy JA, Goyle KB, Reid HL (1977) Treatment of severe intermittent claudication by controlled defibrination. Lancet 1:625
8. Schoop W, Levy H, Schoop B, Gaentzsch A (1983) Experimentelle und klinische Studien zu der sekundären Prävention der peripheren Arteriosklerose. In: Bollinger A, Rhyner K (eds) Thrombozytenfunktionshemmer. Thieme, Stuttgart New York, pp 49–58
9. Hess H, Mietaschk A, Deichsel G (1985) Drug-induced inhibition of platelet function delays progression in peripheral occlusive arterial disease. A prospective double-blind arteriographically controlled trial. Lancet 1:415–419
10. Stiegler H, Hess H, Mietaschk A, Tramppisch HJ, Ingrisch H (1984) Einfluß von Ticlopidin auf die periphere oblitierende Arteriopathie. Dtsch Med Wochenschr 109:1240–1243
11. Gachet C, Stierle A, Bouloux C, Maffrand JP, Cazenave JP (1987) The thienopyridine PCR 4099 inhibits the ADP aggregation pathway of human platelets by interfering with the binding of fibrinogen to the glycoprotein IIb/IIIa complex. Thromb Haemost 58: Abstract 782
12. Katsumura T (1984) Therapeutic effect of ticlopidine for ischemic leg ulcers. Agents and actions. Supplement Ticlopidine: Quo Vadis 15:167–172
13. Prevention of Atherosclerotic Complications with Ketanserin Trial Group (1989) Prevention of atherosclerotic complications: controlled trial of ketanserin. Br Med J 298:424–430
14. Gauthier O (1987) Efficacy and safety of CY 216 in the treatment of specific leg ulcers. In: Breddin K, Fareed J, Samama M (eds) Fraxiparine. Analytical and structural data, pharmacology, clinical trials. Schattauer, Stuttgart New York, p 21 (Abstract)
15. Bounameaux H, Verhaeghe R, Verstraete M (1986) Thromboembolism and antithrombotic therapy in peripheral arterial disease. J Am Coll Cardiol 8:98B–103B
16. Hamming JJ, Hensen A, Loeliger EA (1965) The value of long-term coumarin treatment in peripheral sclerosis. Clinical trial. Thromb Diath Haemorrh (Stuttg) 21:405 (Abstract)
17. de Smit P, Van Urk H (1987) The effect of long-term treatment with oral anticoagulants in patients with peripheral vascular disease. In: Arterielle Verschlußkrankheit und Blutgerinnung, XXX Hamburger Symposion über Blutgerinnung. Editiones "Roche", pp 211–217
18. Kretschmer G, Wenzl E, Schemper M, Polterauer P, Ehringer H, Marcosi L, Minar E (1988) Influence of postoperative anticoagulant treatment on patient survival afer femoropopliteal vein bypass surgery. Lancet 1:797–799
19. Verstraete M, Vermylen J, Donati MB (1971) The effect of streptokinase infusions on chornic arterial occlusions and stenoses. Ann Intern Med 74:377–382
20. Fiessinger JN, Aiach M, Lagneau P, Husson JM, Cormier JM, Housset E (1976) Indications des traitements thrombolytiques dans les oblitérations artérielles des membres. Coeur Méd Interne 15:453–459
21. Martin M, Fiebach BJO (1985) Die Streptokinase-Behandlung peripherer Arterien und Venenverschlüsse unter besonderer Berücksichtigung der ultrahohen Dosierung. Huber, Bern, pp 38–40
22. Bonnet J, Brottier L, Colle JP, Bricaud H (1986) Traitement fibrinolytique des artériopathies sévères des membres inférieurs. Haemostasis 16 (Suppl) 4:90–93
23. Graor RA, Olin JW (1989) Regional thrombolysis in peripheral artery occlusions: In: Julian, Kübler, Norris, Swan, Collen, Verstraete (eds) Thrombolysis in cardiovascular disease. Marcel Dekker, New York, pp 381–395
24. Delcour C, Bellens B, Vandenbosch G, Dereume JP, Struyven J (1987) Long-term follow-up of intra-arterial infusion of streptokinase in acute lower limb ischaemia. Vasc Surg 21:339–343
25. Serradimigni A, Villain Ph (1989) Traitements anticoagulants et fibrinolytiques. In: Rouffy J, Natali J (eds) Artériopathies Athéromateuses des Membres Inférieurs. Masson, Paris, pp 314–330

26. Wilms GE, Verhaeghe RH, Pouillon MM, Dewaele D, Baert AL, Vermylen J, Verstraete M (1987) Local thrombolysis in femoropopliteal occlusion: early and late results. Cardiovasc Intervent Radiol 10:272–275
27. Verhaeghe R, Verstraete M, Schetz J, Vanhove PP, Vermylen J (1979) Clinical trial of brinase and anticoagulants as a method of treatment for advanced limb ischaemia. Eur J Clin Pharmacol 16:165–170
28. Elder JB, Ratery AT, Cope V (1980) Intra-arterial hyaluronidase in severe arterial disease. Lancet 1:648–649
29. Ernst E (1987) Hemorheological treatment. In: Chien S, Dormandy J, Ernst E, Matrai A (eds) Clinical hemorheology. Martinus Nijhoff Publishers, Dordrecht, pp 329–373
30. Lowe GDO, Funlop DJ, Lawson DH et al. (1982) Double blind controlled clinical trial of ancrod for ischemic rest pain of the leg. Angiology 33:46–50
31. Tønnesen KH, Sager P, Gormesen J (1978) Treatment of severe foot ischaemia by defibrination by ancrod: a randomised blind study. Scand J Clin Lab Invest 38:431–435
32. Ernst E, Kollar L, Matrai A (1987) Placebo-controlled, double-blind study of hemodilution in peripheral arterial disease. Lancet 1:1449–1451
33. Stoltz J, Bartel M (1988) Einfluß einer adjuvanten Infusionstherapie von niedermolekularen Dextranen (Infukoll M40) und deproteinisiertem Haemoderivat (Activegin) bei chronisch arteriellen Durchblutungsstörungen im Stadium IV nach Fontaine. Zentralbl Chir 113:1044–1055
34. Stolz JF, Cheraud C, Voisin P, Burdin D, Sheiff F, Laxenaire MC (1986) Association albumine diluée-dextran 40 dans le traitement de l'artériopathie des membres inférieurs par hémodilution normovolémique. Incidences rhéologiques. J Mal Vasc 11:344–350
35. Illingworth CFW (1962) Treatment of arterial occlusion under oxygen at two atmosphere pressures. Br Med J 2:1272
36. Koomen AR (1967) The influence of hyperbaric oxygen in chronic arterial obstruction of the peripheral arteries. J Cardiovasc Surg 8:335–337
37. Hart GB, Strauss MB (1979) Responses of ischaemic conditions to OHP. In: Smith G (ed) Hyperbaric medicine. Aberdeen University Press, Aberdeen, pp 312–314
38. Fredenucci P (1985) Oxygénothérapie hyperbare et artériopathies. J Mal Vasc 10:166–172
39. Coffman JD (1979) Vasodilator drugs in peripheral vascular diseases. N Eng J Med 300:713–717
40. Verstraete M (1982) Current therapy for intermittent claudication. Drugs 24:240–247
41. Porter JM, Cutler BS, Lee BY et al. (1982) Pentoxifylline efficacy in the treatment of intermittent claudication: multicenter controlled double-blind trial with objective assessment of chronic occlusive arterial disease patients. Am Heart J 104:66–72
42. Maas H, Amberger HG, Böhme H et al. (1984) Naftidrofuryl bei arterieller Verschlußkrankheit. Kontrollierte multizentrische Doppelblindstudie mit oraler Applikation. Dtsch Med Wochenschr 109:745–750
43. Trübestein G, Balzer K, Bisler H et al. (1984) Buflomedil in arterial occlusive disease: results of a controlled multicenter study. Angiology 35:500–505
44. Nevelsteen A, De Clerck F, Loots W, De Gryse A (1984) Restoration of post-thrombotic peripheral collateral circulation in the cat by ketanserin, a selective 5-$HT_2$-receptor antagonist. Inter Arch Pharmac Therap 270:268–279
45. Schaub RG, Meyers KM, Sande RD (1977) Serotonin as a factor in depression of collateral blood flow following experimental arterial thrombosis. J Lab Clin Med 90:645–653
46. De Cree J, Leempoels J, Geukens H, Verhaegen H (1984) Placebo-controlled double-blind trial of ketanserin in treatment of intermittent claudication. Lancet 2:775–779
47. Bounameaux H, Holditch T, Hellemans H, Berent A, Verhaeghe R (1985) Placebo-controlled, double-blind, two-centre trial of ketanserin in intermittent claudication. Lancet 2:1268–1271
48. Lassen NA, Larsen OA, Sørensen AWS et al. (1968) Conservative treatment of gangrene using mineralocorticoid-induced hypertension. Lancet 1:606–609
49. Krähenbuhl B, Holstein P, Nielsen SL, Tønnessen KH, Lassen NA (1975) Induced hypertension as a therapy in Buerger's disease (thromboangiitis obliterans). Vasa 4:407–411
50. Martin M, Hirdes E, Auel H (1976) Defibrinogenation treatment in patients suffering from severe intermittent claudication. A controlled study. Thromb Res 9:47–57

## *Commentary*

*Jean-Noel Fiessinger*

In critical ischaemia of the lower limbs, medical treatment is still too often the only alternative to a major amputation, in spite of developing techniques for revascularisation, distal bypass and angioplasty.

### *Thrombolytic therapy*

Thrombolytic treatment has a special place in medical treatment. Often linked with surgery or angioplasty, its aim is the revascularisation of the ischaemic limb. The indications, as well as the methods, vary considerably from one centre to another. Many elements contribute to these differences: the absence of a correct methodological study showing the benefit in terms of amputation or mortality; the diversity of protocols used; the lack of definition of the clinical situations. The treatment is most commonly given intra-arterially, with the thrombolytic agent being administered directly in contact with the thrombus. With low-dose streptokinase (5000 units/hour) and urokinase, vascular flow can be re-established in 50 to 70% of cases [1–4]; when complementary radiological or surgical treatment is possible, the risk of rethrombosis is reduced. However the dangers of this treatment are highlighted by a certain number of recent reports [1, 4, 5]: haemorrhagic complications as a consequence of fibrinolysis, distal emboli resulting from the dissolution of the thrombus, and complications associated with the catheterisation [4, 5]. Overall these are responsible for 20 to 25% of serious complications. Our own experience follows the same direction with a mortality of 3.2% [2]. These results lead us to a very limited indication for thrombolysis. In our experience, it remains a treatment of choice only when other revascularisation techniques are not practicable. The recent obliteration of a distal bypass would constitute an indication of choise for thrombolysis. The demonstration of a localised stenosis after thrombolysis allows for correction of the lesion responsible for the obliteration of the bypass [4]. Better published results, involving very high doses of urokinase (4000 units/min) [4, 6], should not significantly alter this attitude. It is to be hoped that studies conducted with RT-PA will benefit from a methodology cogent enough to establish clearly its place in the treatment of critical ischaemia.

### *Non-thrombolytic medical therapy*

Other than thrombolysis, the aim of medical treatment is to treat critical ischaemia: (1) by preventing extension of thrombosis; (2) by improving the rheology of the blood; and (3) by improving the systemic localised haemodynamic conditions.

Anti-platelet drugs have no place in the treatment of critical ischaemia; by contrast, however, heparin is widely used. In an emergency it has two goals: to avoid the spread of arterial thrombosis, and to prevent venous thrombosis which would compound the ischaemia. A number of open studies [7, 8] have advocated the use of initial heparin therapy in acute ischaemia, in the absence of sensory and motor signs.

To improve rheological conditions is a hitherto classical approach to the treatment of critical ischaemia. Unfortunately, proofs of the efficacy of this treatment are limited. In a randomised study of 42 patients with severe ischaemia [9], ancrod has not been shown to be clinically more beneficial than placebo. Moreover, defibrinating agents are not available in France. The efficacy of isovolaemic haemodilution, despite promising clinical results [10, 11] remains controversial. Its best results are shown in patients with a haematocrit above 50%.

Massive infusions of physiological serum [12] (3 litres in 3 hours) or dextran (500 ml/3 hours) [13] produce a haemodynamic in addition to a rheological effect. They raise the arterial systolic pressure, the cardiac output, the flow and pressure in the lower limbs. Their clinical efficacy remains however to be demonstrated. Any method which raises systolic pressure by the administration of mineral corticoids or angiotensin [14] is open to question.

Vasoactive treatment is widely used, in high doses, intravenously. Unfortunately, mostof the studies concern patients with intermittent claudication and have shown benefit on walking distance only, so there is a lack of proof for reducing the morbidity of critical ischaemia [15].

*Adjunctive measures in the treatment of ischaemia*

There exists little definitive proof of the efficacy for one versus another therapeutic approach to critical ischaemia. The rare randomised studies available to us underline the importance of adjunctive measures; over 40% of patients not receiving specific treatment for ischaemia improve in the course of the treatment defined in the protocol [16].

The primary element of these measures is represented by treatment for pain. Rest pain is usual in critical ischaemia. To reduce this, the patient often sits for some hours provoking lower limb oedema, which aggravates the ischaemia. By relieving rest pain the patient can elevate his leg, the oedema regresses and thus improves the haemodynamics of the ischaemic limb. The relief of pain and the raising of the head of the bed are thus essential elements of medical treatment.

The prevention of further trophic problems involves local care, cleaning, bandaging and grafting – whose importance is emphasised again by the improvement shown in some control groups [16]. Healing of trophic lesions, quite apart from relieving pain, is often the decisive element in the resolution of critical ischaemia. Physical exercise, where possible, can also contribute to the lessening of rest pain.

With the exception of thrombolytic treatment, the rationale for medical therapy of critical ischaemia is unusual. Although there is little direct proof of their efficacy, anticoagulants, rheological and vasoactive medications are widely used. The essential, however, appears to be to gain time in order to allow additional circulation to develop. It is on this basis that heparin by preventing of venous thrombosis, analgesics for rest pain by reverting oedema, and local care of trophic problems have a major role to play in the therapy of the patient with critical ischaemia. The importance of adjunctive therapy, not directly aimed at ischaemia, renders it necessary to evaluate all new treatment against a control group. Equally, it underlines the necessity for angiological services capable of assuring the implementation of these measures.

## *References*


1. Ricotta JJ, Green R, DeWeese JA (1987) Use and limitations of thrombolytic therapy in the treatment of peripheral arterial ischemia: results of a multi-institutional questionnaire. J Vasc Surg 6:45–50
2. Pernes JM, de Almeida Augusto M, Vitoux JF, Raynaud A, Fiessinger JN, Brenot P, Fabiani JN, Murday A, Gaux JC (1987) Local thrombolysis in peripheral arteries and bypass grafts. J Vasc Surg 6:372–378
3. Koltun WA, Gardiner GA, Harrington DP, Couch NP, Mannick JA, Whittemore AD (1987) Thrombolysis in the treatment of peripheral arterial vascular occlusions. Arch Surg 122:901–905
4. Gardiner GA, Harrington DP, Koltun W, Whittemore A, Mannick JA, Levin DC (1989) Salvage of occluded arterial bypass grafts by means of thrombolysis. J Vasc Surg 9:426–431
5. Fiessinger JN, Vitoux JF, Pernes JM, Roncato M, Aiach M, Gaux JC (1986) Complications of intraarterial urokinase-lys-plasminogen infusion therapy in arterial ischemia of lower limbs. Amer J Roentgenol 146:157–159
6. McNamara TO (1987) Role of thrombolysis in peripheral arterial occlusion. Amer J Med 83 (Suppl 2A):6–10
7. Blaisdell FW, Steele M, Allen RE (1978) Management of acute lower extremity arterial ischaemia due to embolism and thrombosis. Surgery 84:822–834
8. Jivegard LE, Arfvidsson B, Holm J, Schersten T (1987) Selective conservative and routine early operative treatment in acute limb ischaemia. Br J Surg 74:798–801
9. Tonnesen KH, Sager Ph, Gormsen J (1978) Treatment of severe foot ischaemia by defibrination with ancrod: a randomized blind study. Scand J Clin Lab Invest 38:431–435
10. Yates CJP, Berent A, Andrews V, Dormandy JA (1979) Increase in leg blood-flow by normovolaemic haemodilution in intermittent claudication. Lancet II:166–168
11. Bailey MJ, Johnston CLW, Yates CJP, Somerville PG, Dormandy JA (1979) Preoperative haemoglobin as predictor of outcome of diabetic amputations. Lancet II:168–170
12. Housset E, Leduc X (1963) Le traitement des artérites des membres inférieurs par les perfusions intraveneineuses de serum physiologique. Presse Méd 71:333–335
13. Amtoft A (1973) The effect of dextran-40 on capillary blood flow and capillary diffusion capacity in the anterior tibial muscle of subjects with intermittent claudication. Scand J Clin Lab Invest 31:263–268
14. Hansteen V, Lorentsen E (1987) Induced hypertension in the treatment of severe ischemia of the foot. Circulation 46:976–982
15. Greenhalgh RM (1981) Naftidrofuryl for ischaemic rest pain: a controlled trial. Br J Surg 68:265–266
16. Cronenwett J, Zelenock GB, Whitehouse WM, Lindenauer SM, Graham LM, Stanley JC (1986) Prostacyclin treatment of ischemic ulcers and rest pain in unreconstructible peripheral arterial occlusive disease. Surgery 100:369–375
17. Jonason TJ, Jonzon B, Ringqvist I, Oman-Rydberg A (1979) Effect of physicla training on different categories of patients with intermittent claudication. Act Med Scand 206:253–258

# Chapter 9

# Mechanism of Action and Clinical Use of Prostanoids

Giovanni de Gaetano, Vittorio Bertelé and Chiara Cerletti



## 9.1 Mechanism(s) of Action of $PGE_1$, $PGI_2$ and $PGI_2$-Analogues in the Management of Critical Limb Ischaemia

Aspirin reduces cardiovascular mortality most likely by suppressing platelet thromboxane $A_2$ ($TxA_2$) generation, despite a variable degree of inhibition of vascular prostacyclin ($PGI_2$) production [1]. This implies that suppression of platelet activatory and vasoconstrictory prostanoids is clinically beneficial and that such a benefit is not hidden by the concomitant reduced availability of prostanoids provided with opposite biological effects, such as $PGE_1$ and $PGI_2$. However, the prominent role of $TxA_2$ does not rule out the possibility that promotion of endogenous $PGI_2$ production or administration of exogenous analogues may have a therapeutic effect in particular clinical situations.

While the physiopathological role of $TxA_2$ could be defined by a suitable clinical and pharmacological model (aspirin efficacy in ischaemic cardiovascular disease) [2], this has not yet been the case for antiaggregatory and vasodilatory prostaglandins. Only a better understanding of their biological and pharmacodynamic effects will indicate the most correct and favourable way for their clinical use.

### 9.1.1 Antiplatelet Activity

The antiplatelet activity of endogenous $PGE_1$ and $PGI_2$ might be regarded as of minor clinical relevance, in view of the already mentioned clinical benefit of aspirin, suggesting a dominant role of $TxA_2$ over $PGI_2$ within the "haemostatic balance".

The supposed physiological control of *in vivo* platelet reactivity by $PGI_2$ has been questioned. Actually, at variance with $PGE_1$, $PGI_2$ is not rapidly metabolized by lungs, so that it might act as a circulating hormone [3, 4]. However, both its rate of entry into the circulation and its plasma concentrations are well below those needed to inhibit platelet aggregation [5]. Therefore, endogenous $PGI_2$ does not differ from other prostanoids recognized as locally acting unstable hormones released on request. On the other hand, the therapeutic use of platelet inhibiting exogenous PGs by continuous i.v. administration may overcome the limits of their local and short-lasting activity.

This clinical chance is theoretically important, since platelet inhibition by $PGE_1$ and $PGI_2$ still represents one of the most powerful mechanisms of suppression of platelet function. In contrast with inhibition of $TxA_2$, which only represents an amplifying pathway of platelet activation, $PGE_1$ or $PGI_2$ are able to prevent platelet response to any aggregating stimulus by increasing intracellular cAMP, a mechanism of action of wide consequences.

Moreover, at variance with aspirin, $PGE_1$ and $PGI_2$ appear to inhibit *in vitro* all the measurable steps and aspects of platelet activation, namely adhesion [6] and spreading [7], shape change [8], aggregation [9], release of dense bodies' and alpha granules' content [10], expression of fibrinogen binding sites [11] and of procoagulant activity [8]. So, also, may $PGI_2$-analogues [12].

All these properties may constitute the basis for the use of exogenous antiplatelet PGs and their analogues in the acute phases of thrombotic diseases, like that following myocardial infarction, or in the advanced phases of peripheral vascular atherosclerosis, in which the vicious circle between alterations of microvascular flow regulating system (MFRS) and inappropriate activation of the microvascular defence system (MDS) could be broken.

The prolonged clinical use of antiplatelet PGs for long-term prevention of platelet contribution to thrombus formation or even to the development of atherosclerotic lesions, may be limited by the occurrence of platelet refractoriness [13, 14]. This phenomenon may be heterologous in nature, thus involving (besides $PGE_1$ and $PGI_2$, which act at the same receptor site) other naturally occurring inhibitors of platelet function, like $PGD_2$ and adenosine [15].

Discontinuous infusions (6 hours daily) of iloprost, however, have been shown to avoid [16] or at least limit [17] the development of platelet refractoriness. On the other hand, iloprost, a 16-methyl derivative of carbacyclin, though provided with a higher *chemical* stability than $PGI_2$, shares with the endogenous molecule a short *biological* half-life; thus frequent intravenous administrations are required. When tested *ex vivo* upon iloprost administration to patients with peripheral artery disease, platelet aggregation is transiently inhibited after both single and repeated discontinuous infusions [16, 18].

### 9.1.2 Protective Effect on Vascular Endothelium

Measured *in vivo* as inhibition of platelet deposition on atherosclerotic lesions in patients with peripheral artery disease, both $PGI_2$ and iloprost antiplatelet activity seems longer-lasting and more marked [16, 19]. Indeed, *in vivo* pharmacological effects other than the antiplatelet one are possibly involved. A protective effect on vascular endothelium could have contributed to this result (see also Section 3.3.2). Iloprost has been shown indeed to prevent hypoxia-induced loss of endothelial function mediated by EDRF [20], a factor of critical relevance in MDS regulation and a pivotal actor in the MFRS.

### 9.1.3 Inhibitory Activity on Leukocytes

Moreover, PGs inhibitory activity on leukocytes [21] and on their interaction with platelets [22] should be considered. This is an important issue: the relevance of the pathogenetic role of leukocytes in cardiovascular disease is supported by epidemiologic observation of their elevated count in the circulation as an index of atherosclerotic risk [23] (see also Section 3.3.5). Polymorphonuclear leukocytes and monocytes not only contribute to thrombus formation but also exert a direct action on ischaemic tissues by releasing several cytotoxic factors. Moreover, there is increasing evidence indicating a reciprocal potentiation between platelet and leukocyte activities, which might influence the site, the dynamic and the extent of thrombus formation and of tissue ischaemic lesions. Because of these properties, activated leukocytes, as a part of altered MDS together with activated platelets and injured endothelium, may cause severe tissue damage (see Section 3.4).

The effectiveness of both $PGI_2$ [24] and iloprost [25] during acute myocardial ischaemia and reperfusion, in fact, was mainly ascribed to inhibition of neutrophil function. $PGE_1$ and $PGI_2$ may inhibit leukocyte chemotaxis by blocking leukotriene $B_4$ production [26]. These PGs may also limit tissue damage by inhibiting lysosomal enzyme release from stimulated human neutrophils, as observed both *in vitro* [27] and *ex vivo* [28], as well as human PMN superoxide production [29].

### 9.1.4 Vasodilatory Activity

The fact that both $PGI_2$ [30] and iloprost [31, 32] protect ischaemic myocardium in experimental models of coronary artery occlusion-reperfusion – even in the absence of major systemic and local haemodynamic effects – questions the relevance of vasodilatory activity of these PGs in limiting the infarct size. A reduced systemic blood pressure might actually lower afterload and thus oxygen demand of myocardium [33]; an increased collateral blood flow might enhance oxygen delivery [34]. Of course, the myocardial model cannot dispel the possibility that the vasodilatory property of these PGs plays a protective role on MFRS (see Section 3.4) of peripheral circulation, maintaining the capillary patency and dilating the lumen of arterioles and larger vessels injured by atherosclerotic lesions.

### 9.1.5 Inhibition of Catecholamine Release

Besides inhibition of leukocyte function, inhibition of catecholamine release from myocardial stores has also been proposed. At variance with $PGE_1$, both $PGI_2$ [35] and iloprost [36] inhibit catecholamine overflow from perivascular sympathetic nerve fibres, thus reducing the release of a platelet stimulus, the beta-adrenergic stimulation of myocardium metabolism, the presence of an inducer of ionized calcium influx across the sarcolemma and of ionized calcium overload into mitochondria.

### 9.1.6 "Profibrinolytic" Effect

Another mechanism of possible benefit in ischaemic disorders is the "profibrinolytic" effect of prostanoids. This was suggested by direct evidence from the use of $PGI_2$ or iloprost in patients with peripheral vascular disease [37–39].

A causal relationship between defective prostacyclin production and reduced vascular fibrinolytic activity was supported by pharmacological studies [40] in healthy volunteers as well as by pathological [41] and pharmacological [42] models of reduction of endogenous $PGI_2$ and of its replacement by exogenous analogues. Iloprost restored a normal fibrinolytic response in atherosclerotic patients with defective fibrinolytic reserve, possibly by replacing endogenous prostacyclin production. Iloprost also reversed aspirin-impaired fibrinolytic response to venous occlusion in healthy subjects.

The mechanism by which prostanoids promote fibrinolytic response is still undefined. Neither tissue-type plasminogen activator release is increased nor the levels of its inhibitors significantly reduced by iloprost [42]. This compound, on the other hand, does not show any direct fibrinolytic activity at least at the concentrations reached *in vivo* [41]. Nevertheless, the profibrinolytic effect of prostanoids might be clinically relevant, since it could help maintaining a normal function of MDS.

While the pharmacological effects related to vasodilatory and antiplatelet properties of prostanoids can explain their rapidly appearing biological effects, the reported long-lasting effect in atherosclerotic patients with peripheral vascular disease still lacks an interpretation. Three day discontinuous infusions of iloprost in patients with *claudicatio* or severe peripheral artery disease reportedly improved functional parameters (*claudicatio* and total walking distances) and relieved pain for at least four weeks, even if this treatment did not affect either calf blood flow [43, 44] or blood rheology [45]. A delayed prolonged clinical benefit is difficult to reconcile with most of the transient pharmacological effects considered above.

### 9.1.7 Cytoprotective Effect

In the last few years a cytoprotective effect of $PGI_2$ and its analogues was claimed as a mechanism of cell preservation. Such an effect is possibly unrelated to the maintenance of a correct MFRS and MDS function but still needs to be better defined. The cytoprotective action of $PGI_2$ first observed on gastric and intestinal mucosa [46] might not be confined to specific cell or organ targets. Biochemical changes induced by prostanoids at the site of both outer [36] and inner [32] cell membranes might improve the injured cell resistance to noxious stimuli. This could limit uncontrolled influx of ions like $Ca^{2+}$ through cellular or mitochrondrial membranes (leading to impaired oxidative peroxidation and loss of energy production); outflow of cell contents, like lysosomal proteases or potentially dangerous mediators (noradrenaline from adrenergic nerve terminals) would also be limited as well as loss of membrane phospholipids and release of fatty acids readily subject to peroxidation.

### 9.1.8 Stimulatory Effect on Cholesterol-Ester Hydrolysis

Besides protecting cells from occasional acute ischaemia, prostanoids could even prevent the progress of atherogenesis before it can lead to chronic ischaemia (due to vessel lumen reduction) or to acute ischaemia (due to thrombotic occlusion). $PGI_2$ stimulatory effect on cholesterol-ester hydrolysis in smooth muscle cell cultures from rabbit aorta [47] may reduce cholesterol accumulation in lysosomal and cytosolic compartment of these cells as well as in their extracellular matrix in atherosclerotic lesions. Cholesterol-ester metabolism was enhanced by $PGI_2$ mimetics also in smooth muscle cells cultured from human atherosclerotic lesions [48], thus reducing cholesterol-ester and triglyceride levels in the cells.

### 9.1.9 Interference with Intimal Proliferation of Smooth Muscle Cells

Besides lipid deposition, smooth muscle cell proliferation and migration into the intima are early phenomena of atherogenesis. Mitogen factors and chemotactic agents are released by platelets, macrophages and altered endothelial cells. Interference with intimal proliferation of smooth muscle cells by $PGI_2$ and its analogues results from inhibition of mitogen release from other cells [49] or from a direct inhibitory effect on smooth muscle cells [50].

Both stimulation of cholesterol metabolism and inhibition of smooth muscle cell proliferation are mediated by cyclic-AMP elevation. Though short-lasting and concomitant only to the administration of prostanoids, this mechanism of action could be reconciled with a delayed and prolonged clinical benefit because of the particular biochemical and pathogenetic targets involved.

## 9.2 Clinical Results with $PGE_1$, $PGI_2$ and $PGI_2$-Analogues in Critical Limb Ischaemia

### 9.2.1 $PGE_1$

*Uncontrolled Studies*

Carlson and Eriksson [51] first reported the effects of intra-arterial (i.a.) infusion of $PGE_1$ (10 ng/kg/h) for 1–3 days to four patients with unreconstructible leg ischaemia requiring amputation. Marked ulcer healing and relief of rest pain were observed and the planned amputation could be avoided. A few years later the same group [52] described the efficacy of a 72 h intravenous (i.v.) $PGE_1$ infusion in eight patients. On the basis of some controlateral improvement observed in patients receiving i.a. infusions of $PGE_1$, a systemic drug effect was suggested, despite the notion that $PGE_1$ undergoes extensive metabolism during its passage in the lungs [4]. The brilliant results reported by the Scandinavian investigators and the usually poor prognosis for limb salvage in patients with unreconstructible arterial ischaemic disease may explain the reason why mainly uncontrolled trials of $PGE_1$ were conducted in the following years ([53, 54]; see also for review [55]).

*Controlled Trials* (Table 1)

The first controlled study of i.a. $PGE_1$ therapy was reported by Sakaguchi et al. [56]. This was a multicentre randomized, controlled, double-blind study in 65 patients suffering from intractable ischaemic ulcer of the extremities – due to chronic arterial occlusion – in whom arterial reconstructive surgery had not been indicated (thromboangiitis obliterans). High-dose (0.15 ng/kg/min, $n=22$) i.a. $PGE_1$ infusion for an average of 24 days resulted in a significantly higher ($p<0.04$) clinical response rate than did low-dose $PGE_1$ (0.05 ng/kg/min, $n=25$) or oral inositol niacinate (control, $n=18$), but only when the latter two groups were considered together ($n=43$). The efficacy of the treatments at the end of the infusions were mainly based on the degree of the improvement in serial photographs of the ischaemic ulcers (assessed by a Committee working under blind conditions). Results were considered clinically favourable in 15/22 patients (68%) receiving high-dose $PGE_1$, in 11/25 (44%) receiving low-dose $PGE_1$ and 7/18 (39%) control patients. The difficulties and complications related to long-term i.a. infusion should caution against generalisation of these positive results.

More recently, two multicentre controlled, randomized studies have been performed with *intermittent* i.a. $PGE_1$ (10–20 µg over 60 min daily for 3 weeks) in patients with severe limb ischaemia (stage III and IV of Fontaine). In the first trial [57] twelve months after the end of therapy, 15/18 patients given $PGE_1$ (83%) vs 9/16 (56%) given a control infusion of ATP showed clinical improvement (relief of rest pain and/or ulcer healing). In the study reported by Trübestein et al. [58] 27 patients received $PGE_1$ and 24 patients received ATP. At the end of the 3-week treatment, analgesic consumption was discontinued or reduced in 14 patients given $PGE_1$ and in 10 given ATP; ulcer healing was improved in 16/18 patients (89%) after $PGE_1$ and in 8/13 (61%) after control infusion. Amputation was necessary in 3/27 (11%) patients receiving $PGE_1$ but in 8/24 (33%) receiving

**Table 1.** $PGE_1$ in critical limb ischaemia

| Author | Design | N. of patients (% diabetes) | Route | Dosage and schedule | Follow-up | End-points | Results | Statistical significance |
|---|---|---|---|---|---|---|---|---|
| Sakaguchi (1978) | MPCdBR | 65 | i.a. | 0.05 or 0.15 ng/kg/min × 24 days C.I. | End infusion | Ulcer size<br>Pain | Reduced by higher dose vs. P + lower | p = 0.039 |
| Böhme (1987) | MPCR | 34 | i.a. | 10–20 µg/1 h/d × 23 days D.I. | 12 months | Ulcer size, pain<br>Stage regression<br>Amputation<br>Death | Negative<br>Increased<br>Increased<br>Reduced | <br><br>n.s.<br>n.s. |
| Trübestein (1987) | MPCR | 51 (25.5%) | i.a. | 20 µg/1 h/d × 3 weeks | End infusion | Pain, ulcer size<br>Clinical stage<br>Amputation<br>Analgesic cons. | Subjective trends of evaluation | |
| Eklund (1982) | PCdBR | 24 (32%) | i.v. | 20 µg × 7 h/d × 3 days (twice, 1 month apart) | 2 months | Ulcer size<br>Pain | Negative<br>Negative | |
| Schuler (1984) | MPCdBR | 120 (60%) | i.v. | 20 ng/kg/min × 72 h (repeated 2 weeks) | 2 months | Ulcer size<br>Pain | Negative<br>Negative | |
| Telles (1984) | PCdBR | 30 (43%) | i.v. | 10 ng/kg/min × 72 h C.I. | 1 month | Ulcer size, pain<br>Amputation | Negative<br>Negative | |
| Jogestrand (1985) | PCdBR | 16 (6%) | i.v. | 2 ng/kg/min × 72 h (repeated 1 month apart) | 1 month | Ulcer size<br>Calf blood flow | Negative<br>Negative | |
| Diehm (1987) | PCdBR | 23 | i.v. | 60 µg/4 h/d × 3 weeks | 1 month | Pain<br>Analgesic cons.<br>Clinical stage | Reduced<br>Reduced<br>Increased | n.s.<br>n.s.<br>n.s. |

C, Controlled; PC, Placebo-controlled; dB, double-blind; sB, single-blind; R, randomized; C.O., cross-over; M, multicentre; C.I., continuous infusion; D.I., discontinuous infusion.

**Table 2.** Summary of the results reported by Schuler et al. (1984) [60]. Ulcers were measured and photographed before infusion and after 2-month follow-up

| Result (% ulcers) | $PGE_1$ (patients n = 57) (ulcers n = 95) | Placebo (patients n = 63) (ulcers n = 115) |
|---|---|---|
| Ulcers healed | 18 | 16 |
| Ulcers decreased in size | 23 | 33 |
| Ulcers unchanged or increased in size | 39 | 39 |
| New ulcers | 5 | 3 |
| Inadequate follow-up | 15 | 9 |

ATP ($p = 0.055$). The authors conclude that, although both ATP and $PGE_1$ had a beneficial effect, a marked trend in favour of the $PGE_1$ group could be observed, not outweighed by the fact that untoword effects led to discontinuation of $PGE_1$ treatment in 3 patients.

The first controlled trial of i.v. $PGE_1$ in patients with ischaemic ulcers due to arterial insufficiency of the lower limbs was reported by Eklund et al. [59]. $PGE_1$ (20 µg/7 times daily for 3 days on two occasions one month apart) was given to 12 patients and saline infusions to 12 control patients in a randomized, double-blind way. One month after the second treatment, no significant difference was noted in ulcer size between the two groups, who both had a wide range of ulcer size and of their variation (f.i. 40% of the ulcers diminished in the control group but the average value showed an overall not significant increase).

This preliminary study was followed by a multicentre, randomized, double-blind trial [60]. This is the largest trial on $PGE_1$ performed up to now. One hundred and twenty patients with arterial ulcers and ischaemic rest pain present for more than three weeks and a mean ankle/brachial index of about 0.5 were randomized to receive either i.v. $PGE_1$ (20 ng/kg/min) for 72 h or a placebo through a central venous catheter. As summarized in Table 2, healing of ischaemic ulcers at the end of follow-up did not differ significantly in both groups. The effect of $PGE_1$ on rest pain was extremely variable and did not differ significantly from the placebo effect. It is noteworthy that one of the 22 centres participating to Schuler's trial had already reported its own negative experience in 8 patients [61]. The four patients who received $PGE_1$ had a significant increase in ulcer size ($p = 0.05$), while the control patients showed no change. Amputation was required within an average of 3 months in all four $PGE_1$-treated patients but only in one of the controls.

No significant improvement of rest pain, ulcer healing, blood flow or amputation rate was observed either in a British or in a Swedish trial. Both studies were randomized, placebo-controlled, double blind. Telles et al. [62] infused $PGE_1$ i.v. (at an average dose of 10 ng/kg/min for 72 h) or placebo to 14 or 16 patients, respectively. All subjects had rest pain and/or ischaemic ulceration due to atherosclerotic occlusive disease of the lower limb and an average ankle/brachial pressure index of 0.5 or lower. One month after the end of the treatment, neither the daily analgesic usage nor the size of ischaemic ulcers appeared to be changed in either group. Seven out of 14 $PGE_1$-treated patients underwent amputation (5 out the 16 controls). No significant difference in pain relief was observed after 1 month follow-up between two groups of 8 patients each, given either i.v. $PGE_1$ (3 ng/kg/min for 72 h) or placebo [63]. In the latter trial the dose of $PGE_1$ infused was relatively low as compared to that used by others.

Fourteen patients with rest pain due to peripheral obliterative arterial disease (without any progression within the last three weeks) were given i.v. $PGE_1$ (60 µg over 4 h daily for 3 weeks) while 9 patients received a placebo. This double blind study [64] showed that – 4 weeks after the end of treatment – reduction of rest pain was noted in 10 patients treated with $PGE_1$ (71%) compared to 4 controls (44%). Five patients in each group showed no change in analgesic consumption but was completely reduced in 7 $PGE_1$-treated (50%) and 1 placebo-treated (11%) patients. A change from stage III to stage IIb occurred in 6 patients with $PGE_1$ and in one with placebo. None of these differences reached statistical significance.

*In conclusion,* anecdotal reports or uncontrolled studies generated enthusiasm and the hope of a new effective therapeutic means to ameliorate the poor prognosis for limb salvage in patients with surgically unreconstructible peripheral arterial disease. Several controlled trials, including the one with the highest number (n = 120) of patients enrolled [60] failed to demonstrate a consistent efficacy of either i.a. or i.v. $PGE_1$ in reducing pain or in ulcer healing. The high placebo response observed in all studies (40%–60% improvement) definitely questions the value of any uncontrolled study and underlines the need for a larger number of patients (than that tested in the trials performed up to now). Short-term i.a. or i.v. infusion – either intermittent or continuous – of $PGE_1$ was considered to be insufficient to achieve a clinical long-lasting benefit; however, long-term i.a. treatment may not be devoid of local complications. Moreover, the question whether $PGE_1$, when given i.v., escapes pulmonary metabolism and reaches the peripheral targets in suitable concentrations remains to be clearly answered.

### 9.2.2 $PGI_2$ (Prostacyclin, Epoprostenol)

The discovery of $PGI_2$, a natural prostaglandin mainly produced by vascular cells and endowed with antiplatelet and vasodilatory activities much higher than $PGE_1$, prompted Polish investigators to test the synthetic compound in five patients with arterial ischaemic ulcers [65]. $PGI_2$ was infused i.a. for 72 h at a dose of 5 ng/kg/min. The results of this historical but uncontrolled clinical study appeared to be particularly favourable: disappearance of rest pain during the second infusion day, ulcers healing in 3 patients within 2 months, the other ulcers markedly improved, the planned amputation postponed.

Similar positive results were observed after i.v. administration of $PGI_2$ and were summarized in 1982 [66]: 65 patients with severe arterial ischaemia experienced long-lasting relief of rest pain (61%) and/or significant ulcer healing for several months (55%). In about half of the patients a positive clinical response could be observed for more than two months. The enthusiam generated

**Table 3.** $PGI_2$ in critical limb ischaemia

| Author | Design | N. of patients (% diabetics) | Route | Dosage (ng/kg/min) and schedule | Follow-up | End-points | Results | Statistical significance |
|---|---|---|---|---|---|---|---|---|
| Belch (1983) | PCdBR | 28 | i.v. | 2–5–10 × 96 h C.I. | 6 months | Pain<br>Analgesic cons.<br>Ankle pressure | Early benefit<br>Long lasting effect<br>negative | |
| Hossmann (1984) | PCdBR C.O.–7 days interval | 12 (50%) | i.v. | 5 × 7 days C.I. | 1 week | Ulcer size<br>Pain | Reduced<br>Negative | $p<0.05$ |
| Cronenwett (1986) | PCdBR | 26 (62%) | i.v. | 6 × 72 h C.I. | 6 months | Ulcer size<br>Pain | Negative<br>Negative | |
| Karnik (1987) | CR | 20 (35%) | i.v. | 5 × 10 h × 5 days D.I. | 4 weeks | Ulcer size<br>Pain | Negative<br>Negative | |
| Nizankowski (1985) | PCdBR | 30 | i.a. | 2.5–5 × 72 h C.I. | 6 weeks | Ulcer size<br>Pain | Reduced<br>Negative | $p<0.02$ |
| Negus (1987) | CdBR | 29 (24%) | i.a. | 8 × 72 h C.I. | 4 years | Ulcer size<br>Pain | Negative<br>Negative | |

C, Controlled; PC, Placebo-controlled; dB, double-blind; sB, single-blind; R, randomized; C.O., cross-over; M, multicentre; C.I., continuous infusion; D.I., discontinuous infusion.

by these studies was not shared by other uncontrolled investigations which failed to show any significant effect of $PGI_2$ treatment [67, 68].

*Controlled Trials* (Table 3)

A randomized, placebo-controlled, double-blind trial with $PGI_2$ was performed on 28 non-diabetic patients with severe peripheral arterial disease (ischaemic rest pain, limited skin necrosis and ankle/arm pressure ratio less than 0.5) [69]. $PGI_2$ (10 ng/kg/min) or placebo were infused i.v. for 96 h. Rest pain was reduced in all patients with $PGI_2$ one day after the end of the treatment and in 7/15 six months later. In contrast, a beneficial effect of placebo could only be found in 3/13 patients (only 1 after 6 months). Analgesic consumption was slightly but significantly reduced during a few days after $PGI_2$ but not placebo infusion. This study was too small to establish whether $PGI_2$ treatment reduced the number of amputations required by these patients.

Subsequently, a randomized, placebo-controlled, double-blind, cross-over study was reported by Hossmann et al. [70]. Twelve patients with stage III-IV according to Fontaine, received either placebo or $PGI_2$ (5 ng/kg/min) by continuous i.v. infusion for 7 days, one week apart. Although this study was essentially of a clinical pharmacology type with measurements of a variety of clinical and biochemical parameters, a significant ($p<0.05$) reduction of subjectively estimated pain was recorded during $PGI_2$ infusion and at least one week afterwards. Ischaemic ulcers and necroses were also reported to heal in 8 patients. In these two European trials relatively high dose of $PGI_2$ or prolonged infusion period were selected in comparison with subsequent studies.

Twenty-six patients with rest pain or ischaemic ulcers (>3 months duration) due to advanced, unreconstructible disease (as judged by arteriography) were randomly allocated to receive i.v. $PGI_2$ (6 ng/kg/min for 72 hours) or placebo [71]. At the conclusion of the study (6-month follow-up) half of 13 placebo-treated patients and one third of 13 $PGI_2$-treated patients had a positive treatment response, as indicated by at least 20% decrease in ulcer size and 33% decrease in rest pain. The positive placebo response, apparent in almost all trials reviewed here, was particularly high in this trial to justify early termination of patients enrollement. Despite the high rate of favourable response, 15 patients were declared treatment failures during follow-up (6 in placebo and 9 in the $PGI_2$ group): this may be justified by the fact that all patients enrolled in this trial had advanced infrapopliteal disease that precluded distal arterial bypass.

Substantially negative was also a more recent study performed on 20 patients with stage III and IV of Fontaine's classification [72]. They were randomized to receive intermittent i.v. $PGI_2$ infusions (5 ng/kg/min for 10 hours on 5 consecutive days) or a conventional vasoactive substance (naftidrofuryl, 600 mg/6 hours on 7 consecutive days). Rest pain and clinical state were judged by means of a score system by apparently unblinded investigators. No better results were achieved with $PGI_2$ than with naftidrofuryl (praxilene).

Following i.a. administration of $PGI_2$, favourable results were obtained in 30 non-diabetic patients with peripheral artery disease without gangrene (half of them were classified as *thromboangiitis obliterans*) [73]. Fourteen patients were non-diabetics randomly assigned to receive either $PGI_2$ (5 ng/kg/min, for 72 hours) or placebo and ulcer healing was assessed on a double-blind basis 6 weeks after the infusion. A significant difference in ulcer area between the two groups was recorded, but previous average duration of ulcers was 40 weeks in $PGI_2$ and 69 weeks in placebo group. On the other hand, there were 8 previous amputations in $PGI_2$ group versus only one in the placebo group, despite random assignment of patients to either group. As in previous uncontrolled trials by the same Polish group, the therapeutic effect of $PGI_2$ treatment was long-lasting.

When compared to naftidrofuryl oxalate (praxilene) i.a. infusion of $PGI_2$ did not show any significant difference in a randomized, double blind study in 29 elderly patients with ischaemic rest pain and atherosclerotic lower limb arteries unsuitable for reconstructive surgery [74]. $PGI_2$ was infused for 72 hours at a dose of 6–8 ng/kg/min through a catheter placed into the common femoral artery (n = 14), while the control drug was given at a dose of 0.02 mg/kg/min (n = 15). The average brachial/ankle pressure was 0.43 and 0.57 in $PGI_2$ and control group, respectively. Relief of pain was observed in 11 patients with $PGI_2$ and 9 controls 24 h after the end of infusion. Long-term results – 7 patients with pain-free foot, 6 with distal amputation and 12 with proximal amputation – failed to show any significant difference between the two treatments.

*In conclusion,* following the widespread enthusiasm generated by early uncontrolled reports, controlled trials showed a therapeutical benefit of $PGI_2$ in some but not all instances. Intermittent or continuous infusion for 72 hours was generally associated with poor clinical outcome, while positive results were seen when the drug was continuously administered for more than 72 hours. There was apparently no advantage of i.a. vs. i.v. infusion (however, these two administration routes were not directly compared in any trial). Similarly, no significant difference was apparent when patients were treated with $PGI_2$ or with a non-prostanoid vasodilator (praxilene).

### 9.2.3 $PGI_2$-Analogues: Iloprost

*Uncontrolled Trials*

Chiesa et al. [75] first associated a dramatic clinical benefit to the use of iloprost, a stable analogue of $PGI_2$, in a diabetic patient for whom amputation of the right leg – because of severe vascular occlusive disease – seemed unavoidable. Although this patient, who was the recipient of a successful kidney and segmental pancreas transplant, was given a broad spectrum of therapy including aspirin, the authors suggested that iloprost prevented the amputation.

*Controlled Trials* (Table 4)

Hossmann et al. [76] had previously reported the results of a randomized, placebo-controlled, cross-over trial of iloprost in 9 patients with stage IV and 1 patient with stage III peripheral artery disease. Iloprost (0.8–2.5 ng/kg/min) or placebo were infused for 12 hours/day for 7 days, one week apart. A significant reduction of subjective rest pain (evaluated by an appropriate staging) was reported during iloprost treatment, while a rather unusual deterioration was seen during placebo infusion.

**Table 4.** Iloprost in critical limb ischaemia

| Author | Design | N. of patients (% diabetics) | Route | Dosage (ng/kg/min) and schedule | Follow-up | End-points | Results | Statistical significance |
|---|---|---|---|---|---|---|---|---|
| Hossmann (1984) | PCdBR C.O. 7 days apart | 10 (70%) | i.v. | 0.8–2.5 × 12 h × 7 days D.I. | End of infusion | Pain (n = 6)<br>Calf blood flow | Reduced<br>Negative | $p < 0.05$ |
| Brock (1986) | MPCdBR | 101 (100%) | i.v. | up to 2 × 6 h × 28 days D.I. | End of infusion | Ulcer size | Reduced | $p < 0.05$ |
| Balzer (1987) | MPCdBR | 112 (34%) | i.v. | 0.5–2 × 6 h × 14 days D.I. | End of infusion | Analgesic cons. | Reduced | $p < 0.05$ |
| Diehm (1987) | MPCdBR | 99 | i.v. | up to 2 × 6 h × 28 days D.I. | End of infusion | Ulcer size | Reduced | $p < 0.05$ |

C, Controlled; PC, Placebo-controlled; dB, double-blind; sB, single-blind; R, randomized; C.O., cross-over; M, multticentre; C.I., continuous infusion; D.I., discontinuous infusion.

**Table 5.** Clinical results obtained with iloprost in patients with trophic ulcers due to severe limb ischaemia

| Author | Diagnosis | Placebo | | | Iloprost | | | P |
|---|---|---|---|---|---|---|---|---|
| | | Total | Responders | | Total | Responders | | |
| | | n | n | % | n | n | % | |
| Diehm | PAOD | 47 | 8 | 17 | 52 | 32 | 61.5 | <0.05 |
| Brock | Diabetic Angiopathy | 51 | 12 | 23.5 | 50 | 31 | 62 | <0.05 |

PAOD: Peripheral Arterial Obstructive Disease

**Table 6.** Clinical trials of iloprost in severe limb ischaemia presented at the International Symposium on Angiology, Toulouse, France, 4–7 October, 1988

| Principal Investigator | Country | Patients (Total n=) | End-points | Iloprost ng/kg/min × /h × day |
|---|---|---|---|---|
| Guilmot, J.L. | France | Stage III–IV (n=128) | • Ulcer healing<br>• Rest pain relief | 0.5–2 × 6 h × 21 days |
| Norgren, L. | Sweden<br>Poland | Ischaemic ulcers not for surgery (n=105) | • Ulcer healing<br>• Death<br>• Amputation | 0.5–2/6 h/14 days |
| Fiessinger, J.N. | France and 9 other European Countries | Thromboangiitis obliterans (Buerger's disease) (n=130) | • Overal clinical improvement<br>• Ulcer healing<br>• Rest pain relief | <2 × 6 h × 21–28 days<br><br>(vs. 100 mg, oral aspirin) |

The results of three randomized placebo-controlled trials have been summarized in a recent publication [77]. The treatment of trophic lesions or of rest pain in patients with peripheral atherosclerotic obliterative disease (PAOD) or diabetic angiopathy was the principal aim of these three studies.

Diehm et al. [78] treated 52 patients (affected by PAOD) with i.v. iloprost (<2 ng/kg/min, 6 hours daily for 28 consecutive days) and 47 with placebo. The same treatment was administered to two groups of 50 and 51 patients, respectively, all affected by diabetic angiopathy [79]. The clinical results of both trials are summarized in Table 5. In both trials, a favourable response to placebo was obtained in about 20% of the patients, whereas more than 60% of the iloprost-treated patients had a positive outcome ($p<0.05$). The summarising report [78] also informs that the clinical benefit of iloprost could be maintained after an average one-year follow-up in the majority of patients, particularly in those with PAOD.

Balzer et al. [80] administered i.v. iloprost (<2 ng/kg/min, 6 hours daily on 14 consecutive days) to 48 patients and placebo to 54 patients with ischaemic rest pain due to PAOD in both diabetic and non-diabetic patients. Twenty three control (42.6%) and 30 iloprost-treated patients (62.5%) were free of pain without any analgesic for at least 5 consecutive days including the first three days after the end of treatment. Despite the high placebo response – especially in patients with PAOD – the difference in favour of iloprost was statistically significant ($p<0.05$).

Several other controlled studies with iloprost in patients with severe limb ischaemia are presently under way. Some of them have been presented at a recent meeting in France (Table 6) (International Symposium on Angiology 1988). The results of these trials, when fully published, will hopefully provide useful information for a better evaluation of iloprost treatment in patients with critical limb ischaemia and for its adequate positioning between reconstructive surgical procedures and amputation.

*In conclusion,* there is presently little information on the clinical efficacy of iloprost in patients with severe lower limb ischaemia, as the principal controlled clinical trials with this drug have not yet been completed and only one has lately been published in final form [76]. Based on presently available information the trials on iloprost appear to have been well planned and conducted in well defined patient groups, with separate trials for diabetic and non-diabetic patients or stratification for diabetes to ensure its equal distribution between control and active treatment groups. Although the inclusion criteria for these trials were not always identical to those of critical ischaemia put forward by a recent Consensus Meeting [81], patients not complying with the recent definition should have been randomly distributed to placebo or iloprost treatment.

## 9.3 Final Comments

The treatment of patients affected by critical limb ischaemia with vasodilatory and platelet inhibitory prostanoids is a relatively new, promising approach to a very severe clinical condition. At present, the available data do not allow, however, any firm conclusion on the clinical benefit of these compounds, although positive results have been observed by several investigators, when reduction of rest pain and/or ulcer healing were considered as clinical end-points. The major problems encountered when analysing the clinical trials performed during the last 15 years on prostanoids and severe peripheral artery disease can be summarised as follows:

### 9.3.1 Inclusion Criteria and Definition of Critical Limb Ischaemia

The inclusion criteria for these trials were not always identical with the criteria of critical ischaemia put forward by a recent Consensus Meeting [81]; in many instances, patients classified as belonging to stage III of Fontaine's classification were enrolled, without any measurement of ankle systolic blood pressure. In several trials (especially those with $PGE_1$) patients with *intermittent claudication* were included, in other trials diabetic patients were not randomized in a separate way and were analysed together with non-diabetic patients. *Thromboangiitis obliterans* (Buerger's) patients too were usually not studied separately with the exception of one trial [56].

### 9.3.2 Treatment Schedule

Both the i.a. and the i.v. route was used to administer the prostanoid drugs. No direct comparison of the two infusion routes has been performed, to the best of our knowledge. The duration of the infusions ranged from 3 to 28 days and was either continuous or intermittent (usually 6 hours/day). These different treatment schedules were not directly compared to each other. In general, iloprost infusions were intermittent and were given for 2–4 weeks, while $PGE_1$ or $PGI_2$ were infused continuously for shorter periods. The question whether the pharmacokinetics of $PGE_1$ permits its i.v. administration without any substantial loss of efficacy remains to be definitively answered.

### 9.3.3 Placebo Effect, Randomization, Blindness

Early trials with $PGE_1$ or $PGI_2$ were uncontrolled. In view of the important placebo effect evidenced by almost all controlled trials with prostanoids, the value of studies without control treatment may only reside in their historical significance. It has been observed that the placebo groups received full standard hospital care and a certain degree of haemodilution induced by blood sampling and saline (control) infusions. As far as controlled trials are concerned, they were usually randomized and double-blind. However, the method of randomization has seldom been mentioned and the resulting groups have not always been compared in respect to important variables before either treatment. It should be mentioned that when compared to a non-prostanoid vasodilator, $PGI_2$ was not superior to it. Moreover, the blindness of a trial where a potent vasodilator is administered seems very difficult to be achieved in clinical practice.

### 9.3.4 Size of the Trial

The number of patients enrolled in any single trial has been relatively small. This should caution against either the possibility that a significant difference could have been missed because of the small sample size or that the occurrence or not of any given end-point in one or two patients might completely change the statistical significance of a trial. In view of the difficulties in running relatively large-scale clinical trials with prostanoids, a *meta-analysis* of all available data would seem to be warranted. More than 800 patients with severe peripheral artery disease were enrolled up to now in the controlled clinical trials with $PGE_1$, $PGI_2$ or iloprost reviewed here (namely, 363 with $PGE_1$, 145 with $PGI_2$ and 322 with iloprost).

### 9.3.5 End-Points

The most common end-points were the relief of rest pain and/or ulcer healing. Several attempts have been made to render these rather "subjective" end-points "objective" (i.e. scales, grading, measurements of ulcer surface). However, the difficulty – already mentioned – to keep the trials double-blind was not reduced by the serious limitation of these "soft" end-points. In only few trials, however, the eventual clinical outcome of the patients (in terms of surgical amputations and death) was also evaluated, but the results were not conclusive.

### 9.3.6 Follow-Up

The follow-up of patients was also quite variable: some trials reported the effects observed already during the infusion of the prostanoids or immediately after the end of the treatment, while others also gave medium or long-term follow-up results. It is remarkable that the reported clinical benefit could be observed in several instances (especially with $PGI_2$ or iloprost) well beyond the duration of the known pharmacological effects of these compounds.

### 9.3.7 Publication of the Results

It is noticeable that very few trials were published in widely diffuse, international, peer-reviewed journals. Such an important clinical issue as the pharmacological salvage of the ischaemic limb should easily find a place in highly reputed journals rather than in the Proceedings of national-based meetings or in non refereed books.

The study by Fiessinger et al. mentioned in Table 6 has lately been published *in extenso* (Lancet 1990, 335:555–557): i.v. iloprost (0.5–2 ng/kg/min for 21–28 days) was well tolerated and had a significantly greater effect than low dose aspirin on symptoms and signs (relief of rest pain and healing of trophic ulcers) in patients with *thromboangiitis obliterans*. In this study the need for major amputation was relatively low and was not statistically different between the two treatment groups.

Sinzinger et al. (Lancet 1990, 335:627–628) have reported that $PGE_1$ synergised with isosorbide dinitrate in reducing platelet deposition and increasing platelet survival time in patients with peripheral vascular disease (Fontaine stage II). The latter drug has been suggested to release nitric oxide, an inhibitor of platelet aggregation and a vasodilator.

*Acknowledgments.* Silvia Falcone and Daniela Spadano helped prepare the manuscript. This work was partially supported by the Italian National Research Council (CNR, Convenzione CNR – Consorzio Mario Negri Sud).

## References

1. de Gaetano G (1988) Primary prevention of vascular disease by aspirin. Lancet I:1093–1094
2. Antiplatelet Trialists' Collaboration (1988) Secondary prevention of vascular disease by prolonged antiplatelet treatment. Br Med J 296:320–331
3. Armstrong JM, Lattimer N, Moncada S, Vane JR (1978) Comparison of the vasodepressor effects of prostacyclin and 6-oxo-prostaglandin $F_{1\alpha}$ with those of prostaglandin $E_2$ in rats and rabbits. Br J Pharmacol 62:105–129

4. Waldhan HM, Alter I, Kot PA, Rose JC, Ramwell PW (1978) Effect of lung transit on systemic depressor responses to arachidonic acid and prostacyclin in dogs. J Pharmacol Exp Ther 204:289–293
5. Patrono C, Preston FE, Vermylen J (1984) Platelet and vascular arachidonic acid metabolites: can they help detect a tendency towards thrombosis? Br J Haematol 57:209–212
6. Higgs EA, Moncada S, Vane JR (1977) Effect of prostacyclin ($PGI_2$) on platelet adhesion to rabbit arterial subendothelium. Prostaglandins 16:17–22
7. Leytin VL, Sviridov DD (1982) A model for studying platelet interaction with cellular and macromolecular constituents of the vessel wall in vitro. In: Chazov EI, Smirnov VN (eds) Vessel wall in athero- and thrombo-genesis. Studies in USSR. Springer, Berlin Heidelberg New York, p 173
8. Ehrmann HL, Jaffe EA (1980) Prostacyclin ($PGI_2$) inhibits the development in human platelets of ADP and arachidonic acid-induced shape change and pro-coagulant activity. Prostaglandins 20:1103–1116
9. Moncada S, Gryglewski RJ, Bunting S, Vane JR (1976) An enzyme transforms prostaglandin endoperoxides to an unstable substance that inhibits platelet aggregation. Nature 263:663–665
10. Karniguaian A, Legrand JP, Caen JP (1982) Prostaglandins: specific inhibition of platelet adhesion to collagen and relationship with cAMP level. Prostaglandins 23:437–457
11. Hawiger J, Parkinson S, Timmons S (1980) Prostacyclin inhibits mobilisation of fibrinogen-binding sites on human ADP and thrombin-treated platelets. Nature 283:195–198
12. Pedvis LG, Wong T, Frojmovic MM (1988) Differential inhibition of the platelet activation sequence: shape change, micro- and macro-aggregation by a stable prostacyclin analogue (iloprost). Thromb Haemost 59:323–328
13. Sinzinger H, Silberbauer K, Horsch AK, Gall A (1981) Decreased sensitivity of human platelets to $PGI_2$ during long term intraarterial prostacyclin infusion in patients with peripheral vascular disease. A rebound phenomen? Prostaglandins 21:49–51
14. Yardumian DA, Mackie IJ, Brennan EC, Bull H, Machin SJ (1986) Platelet function studies during and after infusion of ZK 36374, a stable prostacyclin analogue, to healthy volunteers. Haemostasis 16:20–26
15. Bertelè V, Stemerman M, Shafer A, Adelman B, Smith M, Fuhro R, Salzman EW (1985) Refractoriness of platelets to prostaglandins after infusion in rabbits. J Lab Clin Med 106:551–561
16. Fitscha P, Tiso B, Krais T, Sinzinger H (1987) Effect of iloprost on in vivo and in vitro platelet function in patients with peripheral vascular disease. In: Samuelsson B, Paoletti R, Ramwell PW (eds) Adv Prostaglandin Thromboxane Leukotriene Res, vol 17. Raven Press, New York, pp 450–454
17. Modesti PA, Fortini A, Poggesi L, Boddi M, Abbate R, Gensini GF (1987) Acute reversible reduction of $PGI_2$ platelet receptors after iloprost infusion in man. Thromb Res 48:663–669
18. Darius H, Hossmann V, Schrör (1986) Antiplatelet effect of intravenous iloprost in patients with peripheral arterial obliterative disease. Klin Wochenschr 64:545–551
19. Sinzinger H, Fitscha P (1984) Epoprostenol and platelet deposition in atherosclerosis. Lancet I:905–906
20. Turker RK, Demirel E (1988) Iloprost maintains acetylcholine relaxations of isolated rabbit aortic strips submitted to hypoxia. Pharmacology 36:151–155
21. Belch JJF, Saniabaldi AR, Forbes CD (1987) Whole blood white cell aggregation: a novel technique. Thromb Res 48:631–639
22. Del Maschio A, Evangelista V, Rajtar G, Chen ZM, Cerletti C, de Gaetano G (1990) Platelet activation by polymorphonuclear leukocytes exposed to chemotactic agents. Am J Physiol 258:H870–H879
23. Ernst E, Hammerschmidt DE, Bagge VU, Matrai A, Dormandy JA (1987) Leukocytes and the risk of ischemic disease. JAMA 257:2318–2324
24. Simpson PJ, Lucchesi BR (1987) Free radicals and myocardial ischemia and reperfusion injury. J Lab Clin Med 110:13–30
25. Simpson PJ, Mickelson J, Fantone JC, Gallagher KP, Lucchesi BR (1987) Iloprost inhibits neutrophil function in vitro and in vivo and limits experimental infarct size in canine heart. Circ Res 60:666–673

26. Ham EA, Soderman DD, Zanetti ME, Dougherty HW, McCauley E, Kuehl F (1983) Inhibition by prostaglandins of leukotriene $B_4$ release from activated neutrophils. Proc Natl Acad Sci USA 80:4349–4353
27. Smith RJ, Iden SS (1980) Pharmacological modulation of chemotactic factor-elicited release of granule-associated enzymes from human neutrophils. Biochem Pharmacol 29:2389–2395
28. Fantone JC, Kunkel SL, Ward PA, Zurier RB (1981) Suppression of human polymorphonuclear leukocyte function after intravenous infusion of $PGE_1$. Prostaglandins Leukotrienes Med 2:195
29. Fantone JC, Kinnes DA (1983) Prostaglandin $E_1$ and prostaglandin $I_2$ modulation of superoxide production by human neutrophils. Biochem Biophys Res Commun 113:506–512
30. Melin JA, Becker LC (1983) Salvage of ischemic myocardium by prostacyclin during experimental myocardial infarction. J Am Coll Cardiol 2:279–286
31. Chiariello M, Golino P, Cappelli-Bagazzi M, Ambrosio G, Tritto I, Salvatore M (1988) Reduction in infarct size by the prostacyclin analogue iloprost (ZK 36374) after experimental coronary artery occlusion reperfusion. Am Heart J 115:499–504
32. Ferrari R, Cargnoni A, Ceconi C, Curello S, Belloli S, Albertini A, Visioli O (1988) Protective effect of a prostacyclin-mimetic on the ischaemic-reperfused rabbit myocardium. J Mol Cell Cardiol 20:1095–1106
33. Lefer AM, Ogletree MNL, Smith JB, Silver MJ, Nicolaou KC, Barnette WE, Gasic GP (1978) Prostacyclin: a potentially valuable agent for preserving ischemic myocardial tissue in acute myocardial ischemia. Science 200:52–54
34. Jugdutt BI, Hutchins GM, Bulkley BH, Becker LC (1981) Dissimilar effects of prostacyclin, prostaglandin $E_1$ and prostaglandin $E_2$ on myocardial infarct size after coronary occlusion in conscious dogs. Circ Res 49:685–700
35. Schrör K, Addicks K, Darius H, Ohlendorf R, Rösen P (1981) $PGI_2$ inhibits ischemia-induced platelet activation and prevents myocardial damage by inhibition of catecholamine release. Evidence for cAMP as a common denominator. Thromb Res 21:175–180
36. Schrör K, Funke K (1985) Prostaglandins and myocardial noradrenaline overflow after sympathetic nerve stimulation during ischemia and reperfusion. J Cardiovasc Pharmacol 7, (suppl 5):S50–S54
37. Dembinska-Kiec A, Kostka-Trabka E, Gryglewski RJ (1982) Effect of prostacyclin on fibrinolytic activity in patients with arteriosclerosis obliterans. Thromb Haemostas 47:190
38. Szczeklik A, Kopec M, Sladek K, Musial J, Chmielewska J, Teisseyre E, Dudek-Wojciechowska G, Palester-Chlebowczyk M (1983) Prostacyclin and the fibrinolytic system in ischemic vascular disease. Thromb Res 29:655–660
39. Musial J, Wilczynska M, Sladek K, Cierniewski CS, Nizankowski R, Szczeklik A (1986) Fibrinolytic activity of prostacyclin and iloprost in patients with peripheral arterial disease. Prostaglandins 31:61–70
40. de Gaetano G, Carriero MR, Cerletti C, Mussoni L (1986) Low dose aspirin does not prevent fibrinolytic response to venous occlusion. Biochem Pharmacol 35:3147–3150
41. Bertelé V, Mussoni L, Del Rosso G, Pintucci G, Carriero MR, Merati MG, Libretti A, de Gaetano G (1988) Defective fibrinolytic response in atherosclerotic patients. Effect of iloprost and its possible mechanism of action. Thromb Haemost 60:141–144
42. Bertelé V, Mussoni L, Pintucci G, Del Rosso G, Romano G, de Gaetano G, Libretti A (1989) The inhibitory effect of aspirin on fibrinolysis is reversed by iloprost, a prostacyclin analogue. Thromb Hemost 61:286–288
43. Roberts DH, Linge K, Nixon DP, Chatlani PT, Mc Loughlin GA, Breckenridge AM (1988) The effect of iloprost on calf blood flow in patients with severe peripheral arterial disease. Br J Clin Pharmacol 25:147–148
44. Roberts DH, Linge K, Nixon DP, Chatlani PT, Mc Loughlin GA, Breckenridge AM (1988) The effect of iloprost on calf blood flow in patients with stable intermittent claudication. Br J Clin Pharmacol 25:148–149
45. Ernst E, Marshall M, Matrai A (1988) Does prostacyclin analogue iloprost change blood rheology? Vasa 17:89–91
46. Robert A (1976) Antisecretory, antiulcer, cytoprotective and diarrheogenic properties of prostaglandins. In: Samuelsson B, Paoletti R (eds) Adv Prostaglandins Thromboxane Res 2:507–520

47. Hajjar DP, Weksler BB (1983) Metabolic activity of cholesteryl esters in aortic smooth muscle cells is altered by prostaglandins $I_2$ and $E_2$. J Lipid Res 24:1176–1185
48. Orekhov AN, Tertov VV, Mazurov AV, Andreeva ER, Repin VS, Smirnov VN (1986) "Regression" of atherosclerosis in cell culture: effects of stable prostacyclin analogues. Drug Dev Res 9:189–201
49. Willis AL, Smith DL, Vigo C, Kluge AF (1986) Effects of prostacyclin and orally active stable mimetic agent RS-93427-007 on basic mechanism of atherogenesis. Lancet II:682–683
50. Orekhov AN, Tertov VV, Smirnov VN (1983) Prostacyclin analogues as antiatherosclerotic drugs. Lancet II:521
51. Carlson LA, Eriksson I (1973) Femoral-artery infusion of prostaglandin $E_1$ in severe peripheral vascular disease. Lancet I:155–156
52. Carlson LA, Olsson AG (1976) Intravenous prostaglandin $E_1$ in severe peripheral vascular disease. Lancet II:810
53. Sethi GK, Scott SM, Takaro T (1980) Effect on intra-arterial infusion of $PGE_1$ in patients with severe ischemia of lower extremity. J Cardiovasc Surg 21:185–191
54. Gruss JD, Bartels D, Ohta T, Machado JL, Schlechtweg B (1982) Conservative treatment of inoperable arterial occlusions of the lower extremities with intra-arterial prostaglandin $E_1$. Br J Surg 69:S11–S13
55. Cronenwett JL (1986) The use of prostaglandins $PGE_1$ and $PGI_2$ in peripheral arterial ischemia. J Vasc Surg 3:370–374
56. Sakaguchi S, Kusaba A, Mishima Y, Kamya K, Nishimura A, Furukawa K, Shionoya S, Kawashima M, Katsumura T, Sakuma A (1978) A multi-clinical double blind study with $PGE_1$ (α-cyclodextrin clathrate) in patients with ischemic ulcer of the extremities. Vasa 7:263–267
57. Böhme H, Brülisauer M, Härtel U, Bollinger A (1987) Kontrollierte Studie zur Wirksamkeit von i.a. Prostaglandin $E_1$ Infusionen bei peripherer arterieller Verschlußkrankheit im Stadium III und IV. Vasa (Suppl 20):206–208
58. Trübestein G, Diehm C, Gruss JD, Horsch S (1987) Prostaglandin $E_1$ in chronic arterial disease-a multicenter study. Vasa (Suppl 17):39–43
59. Eklund AE, Eriksson G, Olsson AG (1982) A controlled study showing significant short term effect of prostaglandin $E_1$ in healing of ischaemic ulcers of the lower limb in man. Prostaglandins Leukotrienes Med 8:265–271
60. Schuler JJ, Flanigan DP, Holcroft JW, Ursprung JJ, Mohrland JS, Pyke J (1984) Efficacy of prostaglandin $E_1$ in the treatment of lower extremity ischemic ulcers secondary to peripheral vascular occlusive disease. J Vasc Surg 1:160–170
61. Rhodes RS, Heard SE (1983) Detrimental effect of high-dose prostaglandin $E_1$ in the treatment of ischemic ulcers. Surgery 93:839–842
62. Telles GS, Campbell WB, Wood RFM, Collin J, Baird RN, Morris PJ (1984) Prostaglandin $E_1$ in severe lower limb ischaemia: a double-blind controlled trial. Br J Surg 71:506–508
63. Jogestrand T, Olsson AG (1985) The effect of intravenous prostaglandin $E_1$ on ischaemic pain and on leg blood-flow in subjects with peripheral artery disease: a double-blind controlled study. Clin Physiol 5:495–502
64. Diehm C, Stammler F, Hübsch-Müller C, Eckstein HH, Simini B (1987) Clinical effects of intravenously administered prostaglandin $E_1$ in patients with rest pain due to peripheral obliterative arterial disease (POAD). A preliminary report on a placebo-controlled double-blind study. Vasa (Suppl 17):52–56
65. Szczeklik A, Skawinski S, Gluszko P, Nizankowski R, Szczeklik J, Gryglewski RJ (1979) Successful therapy of advanced arteriosclerosis obliterans with prostacyclin. Lancet I:1111–1114
66. Szczeklik A, Gryglewski RJ (1982) Prostaglandins as therapeutic agents in cardiovascular disease. In: Herman AG, Vanhoutte PM, Denolin H, Goossens A (eds) Cardiovascular pharmacology of the prostaglandins. Raven Press, New York, pp 347–359
67. Pardy BJ, Lewis JD, Eastcott HHG (1981) Preliminary experience with prostaglandin $E_1$ and $I_2$ in peripheral vascular disease. Surgery 88:826–832
68. Vermylen J, Chamone DAF, Machin SJ, Defreyn CR, Verstraete M (1980) Prostacyclin in inoperable ischaemic rest pain. Acta Ther 6:33

69. Belch JJF, McKay A, McArdle BM, Leiberman P, Pollock JG, Lowe GDO, Forbes CD, Prentice CRM (1983) Epoprostenol (prostacyclin) and severe arterial-disease. A double-blind trial. Lancet I:315–317
70. Hossmann V, Auel H, Rücker W, Schrör K (1984) Prolonged infusion of prostacyclin in patients with advanced stages of peripheral vascular disease: a placebo-controlled cross-over study. Klin Wochenschr 62:1108–1114
71. Cronenwett JL, Zelenock GB, Whitehouse WM, Lindenauer SM, Graham LM, Stanley JC (1986) Prostacyclin treatment of ischemic ulcers and rest pain in unrecontructible peripheral arterial occlusive disease. Surgery 100:369–375
72. Karnik R, Valentin A, Slany J (1987) Prostacyclin versus naftidrofuryl. Herz/Kreislauf 1:23–26
73. Nizankowski R, Krolikowski W, Beilatowicz J, Szczeklik A (1985) Prostacyclin for ischemic ulcers in peripheral arterial disease. A random-assignement, placebo-controlled study. Thromb Res 37:21–28
74. Negus D, Irving JD, Friedgood A (1987) Intra-arterial prostacyclin compared to praxilene in the management of severe lower limb ischaemia: a double-blind trial. J Cardiovasc Surg 28:196–199
75. Chiesa R, Vicari A, Mari G, Galimberti M, Di Carlo V, Pozza G (1985) Use of stable prostacyclin analogue ZK36374 to treat severe lower limb ischaemia. Lancet II:95–96
76. Hossmann V, Auel H, Schrör K (1984) Placebo kontrollierte Cross-Over-Studie über die Wirkung von Iloprost (ZK 36374) auf fortgeschrittene Stadien der arteriellen Verschlußkrankheit. In: Trübstein G (ed) Konservative Therapie arterieller Durchblutungsstörungen. Bonn, pp 186–191
77. Oberender H, Krais Th, Schäfer M, Belcher G (1989) Clinical benefits of iloprost, a stable prostacyclin ($PGI_2$) analog, in severe peripheral arterial disease (PAD). In: Samuelsson B, Wong YK (eds) Adv Prostaglandin Thromboxane Leukotriene Res 19:311–316
78. Diehm C, Abri O, Baitsch G et al. (1989) Iloprost, ein stabiles Prostacyclinderivat bei arterieller Verschlußkrankheit im Stadium IV. Dtsch Med Wochenschr 114:783–788
79. Brock FE (1986) Placebo-controlled, double-blind multicenter study to determine the efficacy of $PGI_2$-analogue, iloprost, in diabetics with ulcer and gangrene. 14th World Congress International Union of Angiology, München (abstract)
80. Balzer K, Bechara G, Bisler H, Clevert HD, Diehm C, Heisig G, Held K, Mahofoud Y, Mörl H, Rücker G, Stöveken HJ, Walter P, Wolf S (1987) Placebo-kontrollierte, doppelblinde Multicenterstudie zur Wirksamkeit von Iloprost bei der Behandlung ischämischer Ruheschmerzen von Patienten mit peripheren arteriellen Durchblutungsstörungen. Vasa (Suppl 20):379–381
81. European Consensus on critical limb ischemia (1989) Lancet I:737–738

# *Commentary 1*

*Bernd Müller and Günter Stock*

Critical limb ischaemia (CLI) is the first clinical indication where there are serious efforts to evaluate clinical efficacy and to establish an optimal treatment regimen for the prostanoids $PGI_2$, $PGE_1$ and $PGI_2$-mimetics like iloprost. The pathophysiology of this disease, particularly the nature and hierarchy of events finally leading to the breakdown of peripheral microcirculation and to ischaemic necrosis, is still poorly understood. Considering therapy of CLI, it is certainly not obvious how prostanoids should promote healing of necrosis caused by ischaemia since the main primary cause of the disease, occlusion of large arteries, will probably not be influenced by any drug therapy.

With this background, it is difficult to present a concise mode of action of prostanoids in CLI, and the method of proceeding of the authors, rather to discuss effects of prostanoids on those components of blood and vessel wall which might be related to CLI, is logical.

Concerning the very probable contribution of activated platelets to CLI, the chapter hints at the inconsistency between the rather short-lasting inhibition of platelet activation by prostanoids and long-term therapeutic effects. Here, it might be helpful to remember that there seem to be effects which outlast the $PGI_2$-like stimulatory action on platelet cAMP: $PGI_2$ has been shown to markedly prolong the viability of human platelet concentrates after only a short exposure to $PGI_2$ during the washing procedure [1]. Cotrell et al. [2] demonstrated, that a short infusion of iloprost preserved platelet count and, after cessation of the platelet antiaggregatory effect during iloprost administration, normal platelet function throughout a 3 hour extracorporeal membrane oxygenation. Recently, Lapetina [3] showed in human platelets that following iloprost incubation a ras-related 22 kD membrane protein is phosphorylated and translocated from the cell membrane to the cytosol, thereby offering evidence on the cellular level that processes of transmembrane signalling and enzyme regulation can be influenced by $PGI_2$-mimetics beyond the acute inhibition of platelet aggregation.

The final cause of ulceration and necrosis in CLI is believed to be a compromised blood flow in nutritional skin capillaries, aggravated by a breakdown of microvascular barrier function and perivascular oedema formation [4]. Though the authors mention the relevance to microcirculation several times while discussing the effects of prostanoids on platelets, leucocytes, endothelium, and vascular tone, some additional findings in microcirculatory preparations may further help in understanding the prostanoid's mode of action in CLI. As assessed by intravital microscopy in exteriorized hamster cheek pouch preparations, intravenous iloprost and intra-arterial $PGE_1$ dilate arterioles and venules, increase the density of perfused capillaries, and functionally antagonize vasoconstrictor effects of leukotriene $D_4$ and of endothelin [5, 6]. Experimental microvascular macromolecular oedema induced by inflammatory mediators or by reperfusion after ischaemia is effectively prevented by intravenous iloprost or intra-arterial $PGE_1$ [5]. In a critical ischaemia model in the mouse ear, iloprost significantly limits final ischaemic necrosis and increases perfused microvessel density [7].

According to these findings $PGI_2$-mimetics increase nutritive microvascular flow, counteract increases in microvascular permeability, and correct maldistribution of microvascular blood flow in critical skin ischaemia.

In the case of leucocytes, some additional experimental findings could be mentioned, since they might help to further elucidate the role of $PGI_2$-mimetics in the treatment of CLI. Leucocytes, besides their role in thrombosis, seem to be involved in the pathogenesis of critical ischaemia by showing altered flow properties and aggregation leading to blockade of microvessels [8] and by increased adherence to vascular endothelium followed by endothelial damage through leucocyte-derived mediators and enzymes [9]. Contrary to prostaglandins of the E- and D-series, $PGI_2$-mimetics do not seem to be direct inhibitors of leucocyte activation at therapeutically relevant concentrations [10]. On the other hand, iloprost already at concentrations equivalent to therapeutic concentrations inhibits human leucocyte aggregation induced by activated platelets [11] and prevents FMLP- and $Ca^{2+}$-ionophor-induced leucocyte aggregation in whole human blood [12]. In vitro, iloprost at low concentrations inhibits human granulocyte adhesion to human umbilical vessels [12] and complement peptide stimulated guinea pig leucocyte adhesion to autologous aortic strips [13]. In vivo, intravenous iloprost or intra-arterial $PGE_1$ inhibits increased leucocyte adhesion to predamaged rat mesenteric venules [14].

These findings substantiate the presumption that $PGI_2$-mimetics, in addition to preventing reciprocal potentiation of platelet and leucocyte activation, could beneficially influence pathomechanisms of CLI like obstruction of microvessels and leucocyte-induced damage of vascular endothelium.

The remarks of the authors concerning the mechanisms and clinical relevance of the prostanoid's profibrinolytic effects could be extended by a recent finding in human platelets where $PGI_2$-mimetics inhibited the release of plasminogen activator inhibitor 1 (PAI-1), high amounts of which are stored in platelet $\alpha$ granules, parallel to inhibiting platelet aggregation [15]. It is not clear so far to which extent platelet-derived PAI-1 can impact the overall fibrinolytic potential. It is tempting, however, to speculate that inhibition of platelet PAI-1-release might be the mechanism of prostanoid-induced profibrinolytic effects, which consequently would only become evident in states where platelets are activated and the fibrinolytic potential is decreased by an imbalance of PAI-1 versus plasminogen activator release.

With respect to the clinical results with $PGE_1$, $PGI_2$ and iloprost, one could discuss to which extent $PGE_1$ can be considered a $PGI_2$-mimetic compound like $PGI_2$ or iloprost.

The biological effects of $PGI_2$ and iloprost are believed to be mediated via binding to specific $PGI_2$-receptors on the membrane of target cells (mainly platelets, vascular smooth muscle and vascular endothelium) followed by increases of intracellular cAMP [16, 17]. $PGE_1$, in contrast while exerting its platelet antiaggregatory effect through binding to $PGI_2$-receptors, binds with equal affinity to PGE-receptors of several subtypes from which some are coupled to adenylate cyclase while others use different response coupling pathways, and which are located in different tissues than $PGI_2$-receptors [18, 19]. This results in a pharmacological profile different from $PGI_2$ and $PGI_2$-mimetics in many ways like for example a different profile of cardio- and haemodynamic effects, a different ratio of platelet inhibitory versus vasodilator action, and less effects on the endogenous fibrinolytic potential as compared to $PGI_2$-mimetics [20, 21]. As mentioned by the authors, also the pharmacokinetics of $PGE_1$ differ from $PGI_2$ and $PGI_2$-mimetics; $PGE_1$ being inactivated by more than 90% during one lung passage after intravenous application.

So far there is little systematic information whether the different properties of $PGE_1$ as compared to pure $PGI_2$-mimetics may be of relevance with respect to its therapeutic potential in CLI and to its clinical side-effects. It might be justified, however, to consider $PGE_1$ a prostanoid compound qualitatively different from $PGI_2$-mimetic agents like $PGI_2$ or iloprost.

In their final comments the authors state that on the basis of the present results, a firm conclusion on the clinical benefit of prostanoids is impossible and that, among others, the problem of entirely different treatment schedules hampers comparative analysis of the clinical trials. The most striking difference in treatment schedules was the duration of prostanoid therapy which ranged from single infusion periods of one times 72 hours to 6 hours per day over a period of 28 days (see Tables 1, 3 and 4). In one multicentre, double-blind, controlled study in patients with stage IV PAOD, where healing of ischaemic ulcers was used as an endpoint after 6 hours/day, 28 days iloprost infusion, a careful analysis was made of how therapeutic effects developed during ongoing treatment [22]. It was clearly shown that while a positive trend in ulcer healing could be observed already after 2 weeks of discontinuous infusions, a significant improvement over placebo is seen only after 3 weeks of iloprost infusion and the rate of ulcer healing versus placebo still increases until the end of the 4 week treatment period. Looking at the treatment schedules listed in the Tables 1, 3 and 4, one could conclude that most of the clinical trials might have used too short treatment periods, either in terms of too short individual infusion cycles per day or too few repetitions of infusion cycles, to fully exploit the therapeutic potential of $PGI_2$-mimetics in CLI.

## *References*


1. Blackwell GJ, Radomski M, Vargas JR, Moncada S (1982) Prostacyclin prolongs viability of washed human platelets. Biochim Biophys Acta 718:60–65
2. Cotrell CD, Kapp JR, Stenach N, Fisher CA, Tuszynski GP, Switalska HI, Addonizio VP (1988) Temporary inhibition of platelet function with iloprost (ZK 36374) preserves canine platelets during extracorporeal membrane oxygenation. J Thorac Cardiovasc Surg 96:535–541
3. Lapetina EG (1989) Iloprost causes the phosphorylation and translocation of a ras-related protein. J Vasc Med Biol 1:98
4. Fagrell B (1986) The relationship between macro- and microcirculation – clinical aspects. Acta Pharmacol Toxicol 58:67–72
5. Müller B, Schmidtke M, Witt W (1987) Action of the stable prostacyclin analogue iloprost on microvascular tone and permeability in the hamster cheek pouch. Prostagl Leukotr Med 29:187–198

6. Schulz BG, Müller B (1989) Iloprost antagonizes endothelin-induced vasoconstriction in macro- and microcirculation. Eicosanoids. In Press
7. Müller B, Schmidtke M, Witt W (1989) Effects of iloprost on ischaemia-induced necrosis in the hairless mouse ear. J Vasc Med Biol 1:104
8. Nash GB, Thomas PRS, Dormandy JA (1988) Abnormal flow properties of white blood cells in patients with severe ischaemia of the legs. Br Med J 296:1699–1701
9. Harlan JM (1988) Neutrophil mediated vascular injury. Acta Med Scand Suppl 715:123–129
10. Gryglewski RJ, Szeklik A, Wandzilak M (1987) The effect of six prostaglandins, prostacyclin and iloprost on generation of superoxide anions by human polymorphonuclear leucocytes stimulated by zymosan or formyl methionylleucyl phenylalanine. Biochem Pharmacol 36:4209–4213
11. Pecsvarady Z, Nash G, Thomas P, Dormandy JA (1989) Protective effects of a $PGI_2$ analogue (iloprost) against platelet-induced granulocyte aggregation. Thromb Haemost (in press)
12. Belch JJF, Saniabadi A, Dickson R, Sturrock RD, Forbes CD (1987) Effect of iloprost on white cell behaviour. In: Gryglewski RJ, Stock G (eds) Prostacyclin and its stable analogue iloprost. Springer, Berlin Heidelberg, pp 97–102
13. Fricke D, Damerau B, Vogt W (1985) Adhesion of guinea pig polymorphonuclear leucocytes to autologous aortic strips: influence of chemotactic factors and of pharmacological agents which affect arachidonic acid metabolism. Int Archs Allergy Appl Immun 78:429–437
14. Müller B, Schmidtke M, Witt W (1988) Adherence of leucocytes to electrically predamaged venules in vivo: effects of iloprost, $PGE_1$, indomethacin, forskolin, BW 755C, sulotroban, hirudin, and thrombocytopenia. Eicosanoids 1:13–18
15. Baldus B, Kölsch P, Witt W (1989) Inhibition of PAI-1 release from activated platelets by iloprost and cicaprost. Abstract, 15th World Congr Int Union Angiol, Rome, September 1989
16. Schillinger E, Losert WF (1980) Identification of $PGI_2$-receptors and c-AMP-levels in platelets in femoral arteries. Acta Therapeutica 6 suppl:37
17. Dembinska-Kiec A, Rücker W, Schonhofer PS (1980) Effects of $PGI_2$ and $PGI_2$ analogues on cAMP levels in cultured endothelial and smooth muscle cells derived from bovine arteries. Naunyn-Schmiedebergs Arch Pharmacol 311:67
18. Eglen RM, Whiting RL (1988) The action of prostanoid receptor agonists and antagonists on smooth muscle and platelets. Br J Pharmacol 94:591–601
19. Oliva D, Nicosia S (1987) $PGI_2$-receptors and molecular mechanisms in platelets and vasculature: state of the art. Pharmacol Res Comm 19/11:735–765
20. Müller B, Maaß B, Stürzebecher S (1989) Intravenous infusion of iloprost and prostaglandin $E_1$ ($PGE_1$): cardiovascular profile in anaesthetized rabbits. In: Schrör K, Sinzinger H (eds) Prostaglandins in Clinical Research. AR Liss, New York, pp 401–406
21. Witt W, Baldus B (1989) Divergent effects of iloprost and alprostadil on platelets, blood pressure, and fibrinolysis. In: Schrör K, Sinzinger H (eds) Prostaglandins in Clinical Research. AR Liss, New York, pp 347–351
22. Diehm C, Abri O, Baitsch G et al. (1989) Iloprost, ein stabiles Prostacyclinderivat bei arterieller Verschlußkrankheit im Stadium IV. Dtsch Med Wochenschr 114:783–788

## *Commentary 2*

*Klaus Breddin*

Critical limb ischaemia is a late state of a progressive arterial occlusive disease, usually of atherosclerotic origin and frequently accelerated by diabetes mellitus.

The treatment of critical limb ischaemia is primarily and classically the domain of revascularisation with angioplasty or surgical reconstruction. A possible form of medical treatment which can often be combined with angioplasty is thrombolytic therapy, usually administered in low doses which decrease the risk of bleeding. In about 50% of patients with critical limb ischaemia, at least partial success can be achieved with an acceptable risk using these methods. For the remaining patients, no established treatment exists other than amputation.

Other forms of established medical treatment do not clear occluded larger arteries, nor do they increase the total blood flow. Successful medical treatment in this situation can only possibly improve the homogeneity of the local distribution of blood flow in the ischaemic limb. The pathophysiology of reduced perfusion in critical limb ischaemia, together with the cascade of negative interactive events in the local microcirculation, provide a substrate for limited pharmacological intervention.

It is the essential aim of medical treatment in these critically ill patients to improve nutritive capillary flow in the ischaemic area, thus providing a basis for the healing of ischaemic lesions and the relief of rest pain. Improvements can also be expected from a combined approach with the additional treatment of concomitant diseases such as coronary heart disease and diabetes. Medical treatment in these patients can lead to a limited improvement only.

More specifically, the possible clinical effects of medical treatment may be the relief of pain increasing the quality of life and the stabilisation of the local condition with increased reperfusion of the reversibly damaged tissue leading to a "walkable" leg. Improvement of ulcer healing may permit a more distal amputation.

In a clinical setting where amputation is the only alternative, medical treatment is acceptable even if it produces only partial improvement, for a limited time, in a relatively small percentage of patients. While the final prognosis in many patients probably cannot be altered, gaining time is worthwhile, even if it is limited to months. However, it needs to be said that the duration of improvements in critical limb ischaemia with medical treatment is sometimes remarkable, even though the perfusion parameters do not change at all.

An important factor in the performance and the critical evaluation of clinical trials in critical limb ischaemia is a clear definition of those patients to be included in the trials. Diabetics and non-diabetics should be evaluated separately. Comparability must be reached by randomisation of patients. Clinical end points should be clearly defined, relevant and realistic: for example reduction and healing of superficial ulcers and alleviation of pain.

A placebo is both scientifically and ethically justified, although for practical reasons it is often not possible. Therefore comparative agents can be used which may, at least theoretically, have some positive effect, even though this may not have been proven. Concomitant local treatment should be defined and administered equally to all patients.

The clinical response in such trials should be defined after a relatively short time of treatment, such as two to four weeks. Long term effects should be ascertained by hard end points such as amputation rate or death. Partially objective measurements in this situation are ulcer size and depth. Changes of haemodynamic parameters cannot be expected. At least in principle it would seem to be of interest to use capillary microscopy to evaluate changes in the microperfusion of ischaemic skin areas.

The continuing improvement of revascularisation methods and the increasing opportunities for the successful reopening of small vessels in the limb periphery, combined with antithrombotic drugs and agents to improve the microcirculation, could lead to improved clinical results. A greater and more lasting success can be expected from earlier medical interventions, at a stage where a slowing down of atherosclerosis and prevention of thrombotic complications can prevent the later stages of critical limb ischaemia.

# Chapter 10

# Special Problems of the Diabetic Patient

Wilhelm Krone and Dirk Müller-Wieland



## 10.1 Introduction

Diabetes mellitus is a common disease in the western world, affecting 2–5% of the general population. An important complication of the disease is the development of ulcers and gangrene of the lower limb. The management of these patients is an enormous health problem due to their long periods as in-patient and an amputation rate about 15 times higher than in non-diabetic subjects [1].

Individuals with diabetes are predisposed to foot ulcers and gangrene because of peripheral neuropathy and a high incidence of peripheral vascular disease

(PVD) [2]. Diabetes is an independent risk factor for PVD [3] but is frequently associated with other cardiovascular risk factors, such as hypertension [4], hyperlipidaemia [5, 6], hyperinsulinism [7, 8], and smoking [9]. Hyperglycaemia plays an important role in the pathogenesis of macro- and microangiopathy and is thought to be the major risk factor for the development of peripheral neuropathy [10]. Peripheral neuropathy can result in a loss of sensory perception of foot trauma and therefore may predispose to diabetic foot problems. PVD can lead to gangrene and poor healing of foot lesions. In addition, infection is a frequent complication which aggravates tissue damage of the diabetic foot [11].

In this chapter the special problems of ulcers and necrosis of the lower limb in diabetes mellitus will be discussed. It will focus on the interaction of various precipitating factors causing neuropathic and neuroischaemic foot lesions. On the basis of their differences in pathogenesis and clinical manifestations, the definitions of neuropathic and neuroischaemic limb disease will be discussed. Differential aspects of clinical presentations and various diagnostic procedures will be analysed. Possible therapeutic interventions in diabetic patients with foot lesions will be evaluated.

## 10.2 Incidence and Prevalence

The prevalence of diabetes mellitus in the western world is between 2 and 5%. Of these, 80–90% have type II and 10–20% type I diabetes. Type I diabetes is more common in northern than in southern Europe, the incidence varying from 29.5/100 000/year in Finland to 4.4/100 000/year in France [12]. There is evidence that the incidence of type I diabetes is increasing [13]. During the past three decades the incidence has nearly tripled, and most of the increase has been in the 5–14 year age group.

The prevalence of type II diabetes is age dependent [14], being 2–4% under the age of 50 years and about 8% at the age of 70 years. The incidence rate increases from 5/100 000/year at the age of 35 years to 940/100 000/year at the age over 70. There is evidence that the prevalence and incidence of type II diabetes is increasing over time [14]. Over the last 20 years the rate has approximately doubled in all age groups.

One of the gravest complications of diabetes is the development of ulcers and gangrene of the lower limb which occurs in about 10% of all elderly diabetic patients [15]. Diabetics experience an age-adjusted rate of lower limb amputations approximately 10–15 times that of patients without diabetes [1]. The perioperative mortality rate of these patients is as high as 25% [15], and survival after amputation is poor with only about 50% of patients alive after 3 years [2].

## 10.3 Risk Factors for Diabetic Ulcers and Gangrene

Diabetic patients are prone to develop macro- and microangiopathy leading ultimately to ulcers and gangrene of the lower limb. The predisposition for diabetic ischaemic problems is due to the presence of multiple cardiovascular risk factors, neuropathy, alterations in the immune system, and haematological abnormalities in the diabetic patients.

Several risk factors are thought to play a major role in the development of cardiovascular disease, including hypertension, lipids, smoking, hyperinsulinaemia, and hyperglycaemia.

### 10.3.1 Hypertension

Diabetes mellitus is frequently associated with hypertension [4], in particular patients with diabetic nephropathy have a high prevalence of increased blood pressure [16]. Individuals with both diabetes and hypertension are at very high risk for cardiovascular disease [4].

### 10.3.2 Lipids

Dyslipoproteinaemia, increased levels of cholesterol or triglycerides or decreased concentrations of high density lipoprotein (HDL) in plasma, is a major risk factor for cardiovascular disease [5, 6]. Up to 60% of diabetics have abnormal plasma lipoprotein levels [17]. Patients with diabetes mellitus may have increased levels of triglycerides and/or cholesterol as well as decreased concentrations of HDL [17–19].

Hypertriglyceridaemia in diabetes is caused by an increased secretion of very low density lipoprotein (VLDL) from the liver and by a decreased catabolism of VLDL due to reduction of lipoprotein lipase activity. Hypercholesterolaemia may be caused by a reduced receptor-mediated catabolism of low density lipoprotein (LDL), which is regulated by insulin [20]. The HDL which has a protective role in atherosclerosis may be decreased in poorly controlled diabetes. A major cause for this reduction may be that it reflects elevations of VLDL, since it is a basic tenet of lipid studies that there is often an inverse correlation between VLDL and HDL. Insulin therapy decreases both VLDL and LDL and may increase HDL. In addition, there are alterations in the composition of various lipoproteins which might contribute to their decreased catabolism in diabetic patients [18, 19].

### 10.3.3 Smoking

Smoking is a major pathogenic factor in the development of PVD [9] and patients with diabetes mellitus are high risk individuals when they are smokers at the same time.

### 10.3.4 Hyperinsulinaemia

Epidemiological studies have shown that hyperinsulinaemia is a risk factor for cardiovascular disease. Insulin may be atherogenic by different mechanisms in that it affects lipoprotein metabolism, influences arterial blood pressure and stimulates growth and proliferation of smooth muscle cells [7, 8].

### 10.3.5 Hyperglycaemia

Hyperglycaemia is linked to atherosclerosis and plays an important role in the development of microvascular complications [21, 22]. A major pathogenetic mechanism appears to be the glycolysation of various proteins, such as lipoproteins, vascular proteins, coagulation factors and collagen, thereby altering their function [23, 24].

## 10.4 Definition of Neuropathic and Neuroischaemic Ulcer

A characteristic feature of foot lesions in diabetes mellitus is that there are two distinct diseases: a pure neuropathic and a neuroischaemic ulcer [25]. R 10 A neuroischaemic ulcer is a manifestation of CLI which is defined by the following criteria: (1) ulceration or gangrene at the foot, or persistently recurring rest pain requiring regular analgesia for more than two weeks, plus (2) absence of ankle pulses. A pure neuropathic foot lesion can be characterized by an ulceration or gangrene secondary to peripheral neuropathy, but in the presence of ankle pulses. Patients with purely neuropathic ulcers should be clearly differentiated from those with neuroischaemic lesions because the management of the patient will be different.

## 10.5 Pathogenesis of Diabetic Ulcer and Gangrene

Peripheral neuropathy and ischaemia secondary to arterosclerosis predisposes the diabetic patient to a variety of foot lesions. The pathogenesis of the neuroischaemic ulcer and the pure neuropathic ulcer will be discussed. However, clinically often a combination of both diseases is found.

### 10.5.1 Neuroischaemic Ulcer

In CLI there is thought to be a breakdown of microvascular flow regulation, as described in Chapter 3. In diabetic patients with CLI these changes are amplified and generally lead to more serious disease than in non-diabetic patients. In particular, due to the metabolic alterations in diabetes aggregation of red blood cells and platelets is aggravated, the damage to endothelial cells and white blood cells is greatly enhanced [26]. The impairment of a variety of white blood cell functions including chemotaxis, phagocytosis, bacterial adherence and opsonisation predisposes the diabetics to infection [27].

A crucial feature of all forms of diabetes is that, in addition to fundamental changes in blood glucose levels, there are substantial alterations in the composition and properties of the blood. Thus, changes in fibrinolytic activity, plasminogen and tissue plasminogen activator inhibitor concentrations, prostacyclin synthesis and various plasma proteins, such as fibrinogen and albumin, have been described [26].

Tissue necrosis is often caused by minor trauma, resulting from constant pressure from tight ill-fitting shoes. Decreased perception of trivial injuries due to concomitant presence of sensory neuropathy might aggrevate this problem.

There is a poor healing response because of the ischaemia leading to indolent ulcerations. Minor trauma is often followed by infection [25].

### 10.5.2 Neuropathic Ulcer

Peripheral neuropathy [28] has a high prevalence in diabetic patients. The distal symmetric diabetic polyneuropathy, which is the most common form of diabetic neuropathy, involves sensory, motor, and autonomic nerve fibres. The sensory impairment is characterized by reduced sensation of pain and temperature, numbness and parasthaesia which may be painful. As a consequence, diabetic patients with neuropathy may not be able to notice small thermal trauma, pressure from poorly fitting shoes, and other trauma [2, 25, 29]. This can result in calluses, ulceration, gangrene, and infection. Motor nerve defects may cause foot deformities and a pressure maldistribution on the plantar surface of the foot [25, 29]. Deformities are important predisposing factors in foot lesions. Local consequences of autonomic abnormalities include loss of sweating, dry fissured skin and vasomotor instability with increases in arteriovenous shunting which may possibly lead to capillary ischaemia [30].

### 10.5.3 Small Vessel Disease

There is considerable controversy among diabetologists as to the real importance of small vessel disease [31]. There is undoubtedly evidence showing a thickening of the capillary wall in the diabetic foot but the capillary lumen is not reduced. Although there is no evidence of an occlusive microvascular disease in diabetic patients, there may be functional abnormalities of the capillaries. Functional abnormalities of the capillary wall may contribute to the development and progression of both diseases, the neuropathic and neuroischaemic ulcer, but their relevance to clinical events remains to be determined.

## 10.6 Clinical Presentation

The main clinical features of neuropathic ulcers, compared with those of neuroischaemic ulcers are summarized in Table 1.

**Table 1.** Clinical features of diabetic foot ulcers

| Neuropathic ulcer | Neuroischaemic ulcer |
|---|---|
| Palpable pulses | Absence of pulses |
| Painless | Painful |
| Usually sited over pressure point | No specific site |
| Increase in total blood flow | Decrease in total blood flow |
| Callus + + | Minimal granulation |
| Pressure Index >1.1 | Pressure index <1.1 |

### 10.6.1 Neuroischaemic Ulcer

Neuroischaemic ulcers in contrast to neuropathic ulcers in diabetic patients are characterized by absence of pulses and are usually painful. The main features of PVD in the diabetic leg is that it is diffuse and mainly found in arterial vessels below the knee. A typical arteriogram in diabetic patients with tissue necrosis in the foot shows an occlusion at the trifurcation so that the distal vessels are not shown.

### 10.6.2 Neuropathic Ulcer

Classical neuropathic lesions occur on the plantar surface of the foot. In contrast to the neuroischaemic foot, pulses are palpable, veins can be dilated, and the skin is warm. The anhidrosis of the skin as a consequence of sympathic denervation predisposes to the development of dry skin, fissures, and infections. Repetitive high vertical and shear forces lead to callus formation on the plantar surface of the foot. The abnormally high forces are determined by structural abnormalities which can be acquired or caused by congenital deformities. Neuropathy leads to bone and joint disorganisation which results in increased pressure and friction on bony protuberances. Eventually the callus breaks down with inflammatory autolysis leading to the neuropathic ulceration. Acute mechanical, thermal or chemical injuries also lead to ulceration but are a less frequent cause of tissue necrosis than the classical plantar ulcer. Acute trauma rarely is the cause for an ulceration in the diabetic patient.

### 10.6.3 Diabetic Osteopathy and Neuroarthropathy

Osseous manifestations of the diabetic foot [25, 29, 32] can affect primarily the bone, called diabetic osteopathy, or the joints called neuroarthropathy. Diabetic osteopathy is most frequently present as resorptive zones in the phalanges, but individual lesions are most severe in the metatarsal and tarsal bone. The earliest radiographic signs of neuroarthropathy is soft tissue swelling and joint effusion, followed by subchondral lucency, mild subluxations, small infarctions, or overt juxta-articular fractures. The alterations might progress and deteriorate resulting in bony fragmentation, further fractures, and osseous spicules within the synovium. Healing may produce periosteal and endochondral new bone formation, which can have a sclerotic appearance to juxta-articular bone. These destructions can lead to gross deformities of the foot, particularly the rocker bottom deformity, in which there is displacement of the subluxation of the tarsus downwards, and the medial convexity, which results from displacement of the talonavicular joint or from tarsometatarsal dislocation [25].

### 10.6.4 Infection

Infection is present in the majority of foot ulcers and is a frequent precursor to amputation. Typically, foot infection occurs with multiple organisms, both aerobic and anaerobic [11]. Bacteria can enter diabetic ulcers secondary to fissures, ingrowing toe-nails and interdigital fungal infection. Diabetic foot infections may not cause systemic toxicity, but the foot infection can precipitate ketoacidosis or hyperosmolar coma, even in the well controlled diabetic patient.

Infection may lead to in situ thrombosis of digital vessels. This may result in digital necrosis. Soft tissue abscesses frequently affect the plantar anatomical spaces of the foot. The most common sites of osteomyelitis in the diabetic foot are the first, fifth and second rays [32]. Calcaneal involvement may also occur but the remaining tarsal bones are infrequently affected. Osteomyelitis occurs at a solitary site in the majority of patients. The presence of marked soft tissue swelling or sequestrum formation may assist in identifying superimposed infection. Knowledge of the presence and extent of soft tissue involvement is important in order to avoid or properly determine the level of amputation.

One of the most difficult challenges of radiologic methods is to accurately distinguish between neuroarthropathy and superimposed bone or soft tissue infection. Conventional radiographs as well as a variety of scintigraphic techniques play a major role in the differential diagnosis of these alterations. Promising early results have also been obtained using computer tomography and more recently magnetic resonance imaging, although the ultimate role of these methods awaits further experience.

## 10.7 Investigation of the Diabetic Foot

The clinical examination should include assessment of the colour of the foot, deformity, oedema, callus, and the position of ulcers. Checking of pulses is the crucial method of investigation and should be considered together with skin temperature, skin moistness and the presence or absence of oedema. The neuroischaemic foot may be cold, but in the presence of autonomic neuropathy the foot may be warm. Neurological assessment should include knee and ankle reflexes, together with measurements of temperature and vibration thresholds. For evaluation of CLI in the diabetic patient further investigations are blood pressure measurements, Doppler- and Duplex sonography, transcutaneous oxygen pressure measurements, x-ray of the foot and arteriography. The validities of these procedures which are described in detail in Chapter 4 are discussed in respect of the diabetic patient.

Most ischaemics with absent pulses have a pressure index below 1.0 but there are others with a high pressure index due to arterial calcification [33]. In these cases the clinician can use Doppler sonography to assess arterial stenosis or occlusion. If available, there are several newer techniques which might be helpful in the investigation of microcirculation, such as transcutanous oxygen mapping (tc PO2), capillaroscopy and laser-Doppler flowmetry. The value of these methods in the investigation of ischaemic limb disease in patients with diabetes mellitus is still in debate. Recently it has been reported that transcutaneous oxygen mapping might be helpful to predict tissue healing and to plan the site and timing of amputation [34].

However, the only certain way to determine whether there is a stenosis causing CLI is to use arteriography. In the neuroischaemic foot, arteriography should be performed in all cases. The majority of neuropathic ulcers can be healed with conservative measures alone but if the ulcer proves indolent arteriography should be performed. However, it should be considered that due to the high prevalence of diabetic nephropathy, arteriography may be associated with an increased risk of developing renal failure.

## 10.8 Management of Patients with Diabetic Ulcers and Gangrene

### 10.8.1 General Management

Compared with non-diabetics an even higher proportion of diabetic patients with critical limb ischaemia have coexistent cardiovascular diseases and risk factors, such as coronary heart disease, disease of the carotids, hypertension, heart failure, renal disease, hyperlipidaemia and hyperglycaemia. Similar to non-diabetic patients coexisting diseases and risk factors have to be treated (see Chapter 4).

In diabetic patients blood sugar levels should be normalized as far as possible. Although there are no controlled prospective studies there is common agreement
R 11 that blood glucose concentrations should be at least less than 200 mg/dl. Practically all patients with critical limb ischaemia should be converted to insulin. Several injections may be necessary to reach this target.

Since patients with hyperglycaemia are often dehydrated, they should be rehydrated. Oedema in patients with diabetic foot lesions should be treated with diuretics in order to improve microcirculation by reducing pressure on nutritive capillaries. Many patients suffer from diabetic nephropathy. This should be considered when angiography is planned. The metabolic abnormalities should be assessed and treated before and during general anaesthesia and surgery.

### 10.8.2 Management of the Diabetic Foot

Patients with diabetes mellitus are more prone to the development of foot infections and sepsis of the foot is a major cause of limb loss in diabetics [35]. The infections are polymicrobial with anaerobes being frequently present. Whether there are any benefits of antibiotic treatment is still controversial and might depend on the timing of treatment. It is suggested that systemic antibiotic administration is not used routinely in all patients, especially those with simple flat superficial ulcers, to avoid inducing bacterial resistance. However, if there is any clinical evidence of local or systemic infection and if deeper ulcers with possible fistulae are present, culture swabs should be taken and antibiotic treatment should be initiated immediately.

Patients with purely neuropathic disease should be clearly differentiated from those with ischaemic disease because the management of the patients will be different. About 90% of pure neuropathic ulcers can be healed with rest and regular removal of callous tissue [25, 36–38]. Simple dry daily dressings are required. Redistribution of the high vertical and shear forces can be achieved by plaster
R 12 casts [36], or moulded insoles of shoes [37]. If this does not achieve healing angiography may be necessary. Treatment of ulcerations on the neuroischaemic foot consists of two parts: conservative treatment, and revascularization.

Conservative treatment comprises rest, relief of pain, reduction of oedema, removal of necrotic tissue and daily dry dressings and wide fitting shoes. The foot should be placed in the lowest possible position without inducing or aggravating oedema. Angiography is necessary to investigate arteries of the feet and plan revascularisation.

Bypass surgery and percutaneous transluminal angioplasty (PTA) are possible in a smaller proportion of diabetics than non-diabetics with CLI because the disease is more distal [25, 36]. With advancing catheter techniques, relief of ischaemia is being achieved by arterial reconstruction down to the foot vessels and by angioplasty of the popliteal and calf vessels.

### 10.8.3 Amputations

Amputation rates in diabetic patients are about 15 times higher than in non-diabetics [1]. It should be stressed that an amputation should not be performed without having angiography to exclude the possibility of either percutaneous transluminal angioplasty or surgical reconstruction. A trial of pharmacotherapy should always be considered though none of the existing agents has been adequately tested in this context. Amputations in diabetic patients should be performed only where adequate arrangements exist for full rehabilitation.

### 10.8.4 Primary Pharmacotherapy

There is no evidence available for the efficacy of anticoagulants, antiplatelet drugs, vasoactive drugs or fibrinogen lowering drugs in the treatment of either neuroischaemic or neuropathic ulcers in diabetic patients. Recently, clinical studies provide evidence that prostanoids might be effective in diabetic and non-diabetic patients with critical limb ischaemia; for details see Chapter 9.

There are no controlled clinical trials in diabetic ulcerations showing the benefit of isovolaemic haemodilution alone in critical ischaemia. Since diabetic patients are often dehydrated they should be rehydrated. If the haematocrit remains over 50 despite rehydration, haemodilution may be considered.

## 10.9 Preventive Treatment

Education of diabetic patients is important to prevent development and recurrence of ulcers and gangrene [2, 25, 36, 39, 40]. Prophylactic measures include the provision of suitable footwear and chiropody. Patients should wash and inspect their feet daily and report any calluses, corns, blisters or ulcerations to the physician. Patients should never try to treat the lesions at home. New shoes should never be worn for more than one or two hours a day. Diabetic patients with peripheral vascular disease or neuropathy should never walk barefoot.

The direct cost of an amputation including hospitalisation, surgery and rehabilitation is enormous. It is estimated that over 50% of the amputations within the diabetic population could be prevented by reducing risk factors for diabetic ulcers and improving foot-care [2].

**Table 2.** Targets for metabolic control

| | Degree of diabetic control | | |
|---|---|---|---|
| | Good | Acceptable | Poor |
| Blood glucose mg/dl (mmol/l) | | | |
| Fasting | 80–120 (4.4–6.7) | <140 (<7.8) | >140 (>7.8) |
| Post-prandial | 80–160 (4.4.–8.9) | <180 (<10) | >180 (>10) |
| $HbA_1$[a] (%) | <8 | <9.5 | >9.5 |
| Urine glucose (%) | 0 | <0.5 | >0.5 |
| Total cholesterol mg/dl (mmol/l) | <200 (<5.2) | <250 (<6.5) | >250 (>6.5) |
| HDL-cholesterol mg/dl (mmol/l) | >40 (>1.1) | >35 (>0.9) | <35 (<0.9) |
| Fasting triglycerides mg/dl (mmol/l) | <150 (<1.7) | <200 (<2.2) | >200 (>2.2) |
| Body mass index ♂ | <25 | <27 | >27 |
| ♀ | <24 | <26 | >26 |

[a] Multiply by 0.8 for $HbA_{1c}$
Proposal of the European NIDDM Policy Group

Risk factors for peripheral vascular disease and neuropathy should be treated vigorously. Risk factors to be considered are hyperlipidaemia, hypertension, hyperglycaemia and hyperinsulinaemia. Smoking is an even more adverse risk factor in diabetic patients than in non-diabetics, and patients should be encouraged to give up smoking. Table 2 shows the targets for optimal control of blood glucose and plasma lipids.

These targets have to be individualized according to age, cardiovascular complications and other clinical aspects.

There are convincing studies demonstrating that improved foot care reduces the frequency of amputations in diabetic patients [39, 40]. Therefore, all patients with diabetes should learn to examine and care for their feet by themselves. If a patient is not able to do this a family member or others should be educated to take care of the patients feet. Nurses and doctors must also be educated in special foot-care programs to prevent diabetic foot complications. The education strategies should concentrate on the identification of high-risk patients, performance of regular foot examinations, and assurance of follow-up according to risk.

R 14 No one person can carry out total care of the diabetic foot. This needs a team approach [39]. Close liaison is necessary between the diabetologist and vascular and orthopaedic surgeons who should work closely with the podiatrist, nurse and shoe fitter.

## 10.10 Conclusion

Lower limb amputations in patients with diabetes mellitus are 15 times higher than in people without diabetes, and 50% of all amputations are performed on diabetics. In diabetic patients one has to differentiate between two different diseases: neuroischaemic and neuropathic ulcers. A pure neuropathic foot lesion is characterized by an ulceration or gangrene but with the presence of foot (ankle) pulses, and the lesions will heal with routine conservative management. The neuroischaemic ulcer, however, is a manifestation of CLI, i.e. with absent palpable pulses.

Contrary to non-diabetic patients the lesions of CLI in diabetics are more diffuse. Therefore, PTA and bypass surgery is less frequently performed. However, before major amputation is undertaken, angiography should always be performed as there may be a possibility for revascularization.

There are no definite data available showing a proven effect of anticoagulants, antiplatelet drugs, or other vasoactive pharmacotherapy on the progression of ulcers and gangrene in patients with diabetes mellitus. Clinical trials appear to provide evidence indicating that prostanoids might be effective in diabetics with CLI and therefore may be considered in patients unsuitable for reconstructive surgery or PTA, except in those who require immediate amputation.

The successful prevention and management of diabetic foot disease requires a close co-operation between different disciplines familiar with problems of the diabetic patient.

## References

1. Most RS, Sinnock P (1983) The epidemiology of lower extremity amputations in diabetic individuals. Diabetes Care 6:87–91
2. Bild DE, Selby JV, Sinnock P, Browner WS, Braveman P, Schowstack JA (1989) Lower-extremity amputation in people with diabetes mellitus. Epidemiology and prevention. Diabetes Care 12:24–31
3. Brand FN, Abbott RD, Kannel WB (1989) Diabetes, intermittent claudication, and risk of cardiovascular events. The Framingham Study. Diabetes 38:504–509
4. Members of the Working Group on Hypertension in Diabetes (1987) Statement on hypertension in diabetes. Diabetes Care 10:764–776
5. Assmann G, Schulte H (1988) The Prospective Cardiovascular Münster (PROCAM) Study: prevalence of hyperlipidemia in persons with hypertension and/or diabetes mellitus and the relationship to coronary heart disease. Amer Heart J 116, part 2:1713–1724
6. Study Group, European Atherosclerosis Society (1988) The recognition and management of hyperlipidemia in adults: a policy statement of the European Atherosclerosis Society. Amer Heart J 9:571–600
7. Stout RW (1979) Diabetes and atherosclerosis: the role of insulin. Diabetologia 167:141–150
8. Wirth A, Krone W (1988) Insulin: ein kardiovasculärer Risikofaktor. Dtsch Med Wochenschr 113:1250–1254
9. Kannel WB, McGee DL (1985) Update on some epidemiologic features of intermittent claudication: the Framingham Study. J Amer Geriatr Soc 33:13–18
10. Hatary Y (1987) Diabetic peripheral neuropathy. Ann Intern Med 107:546–559

11. Louie TJ, Artlett JG, Tally FP (1976) Aerobic and anaerobic bacteria in diabetic foot ulcers. Ann Intern Med 85:461–463
12. Krolewski AS, Warram JH, Rand LI, Kahn CR (1987) Epidemiologic approach to the etiology of type I diabetes mellitus and its complications. N Engl J Med 317:1390–1398
13. Bingley PJ, Gale EAM (1989) Rising incidence of IDDM in Europe. Diabetes Care 12:289–295
14. Krolewski AS, Warram JH (1985) Epidemiology of diabetes mellitus. In: Marble A, Krall LP, Bradley RF, Christlieb AR, Soeldner JS (eds) Joslin's diabetes mellitus, 12th ed. Philadelphia, Lea & Febiger, pp 12–42
15. Gutman M, Kaplan O, Skornick Y, Klausner JM, Lelcuk S, Rozin RR (1987) Gangrene of the lower limbs in diabetic patients: a malignant complication. Am J Surg 154:305–308
16. Mogensen CE (1988) Therapeutic interventions in nephropathy of IDDM. Diabetes Care 11 (suppl 1):10–15
17. Ganda OP (1985) Pathogenesis of macrovascular disease including the influence of lipids. In: Marble A, Krall LP, Bradley RF, Christlieb AR, Soeldner JS (eds) Joslin's diabetes mellitus, 12th ed. Philadelphia, PA, Lea & Febiger, pp 217–250
18. Howard BV (1987) Lipoprotein metabolism in diabetes mellitus. J Lipid Res 28:613–628
19. Kostner GM, Karachi I (1988) Lipoprotein alterations in diabetes mellitus. Diabetologia 31:717–722
20. Krone W, Nägele H, Behnke B, Greten H (1988) Opposite effects of insulin and catecholamines on LDL-receptor activity in human mononuclear leukocytes. Diabetes 37:1386–1391
21. Jarrett RJ, Keen H, Chakrabati R (1982) Diabetes, hyperglycemia and arterial disease. In: Keen H, Jarrett J (eds) Complications of diabetes, 2nd ed. London, Edward Arnold, Ltd, pp 179–203
22. Klaff LJ, Palmer JP (1986) Risk for developing cardiovascular risk factors: risk for glucose intolerance. Cardiol Clin 4:67–73
23. Brownly M, Cerami A (1981) The biochemistry of the complications of diabetes mellitus. Ann Rev Biochem 50:385–432
24. Brownly M, Cerami A, Vlassara H (1988) Advanced glycosilation endproducts in tissue in the biochemical basis of diabetic complications. New Engl J Med 318:1315–1321
25. Edmonds ME (1986) The diabetic foot: pathophysiology and treatment. Clin Endocrinol Metab 15:899–916
26. Colwell JA, Lopes-Virella MF (1988) A review of the development of large-vessel disease in diabetes mellitus. Am J Med 85 (Suppl):113–118
27. Cooppan R (1985) Infection in diabetes. In: Marble A, Krall LP, Bradley RF, Christlieb AR, Soeldner JS (eds) Joslin's diabetes mellitus, 12th ed. Philadelphia, Lea & Febiger, pp 737–747
28. Strian F (1986) Autonome und sensomotorische Diabetesneuropathie – diagnostische und klassifikatorische Probleme. In: Strian F, Haslbeck M (eds) Autonome Neuropathie. Springer, pp 3–14
29. Möller A, Haslbeck M (1986) Trophische Störungen. In: Strian F, Haslbeck M (eds) Autonome Neuropathie. Springer, pp 153–170
30. Edmonds ME (1986) The neuropathic foot in diabetes. Part I: Blood flow. Diabetic Medicine 3:111–115
31. LoGerfo FW, Coffman JD (1984) Vascular and microvascular disease of the foot in diabetes. N Engl J Med 311:1615–1619
32. Zlathin MB, Pathrin M, Sartoris DJ, Resmick D (1987) The diabetic foot. Radiol Clin North Am 25:1095–1105
33. Apelqvist J, Castenfors J, Larsson J, Stinstrom A, Agardh C-D (1989) Prognostic value of systolic ankle and toe blood pressure levels in outcome of diabetic foot ulcer. Diabetes Care 12:373–378
34. Rhodes GR, Skudder P Jr (1986) Salvage of ischemic diabetic foot: role of transcutaneous oxygen mapping and multiple configuration of in situ bypass. Am J Surg 152:165–171
35. Scher K, Steele FJ (1988) The septic foot in patients with diabetes. Surgery 104:661–666
36. Levin ME (1987) The diabetic foot: pathophysiology, evaluation, and treatment. In: Levin WM, O'Neal LW (eds) The diabetic foot, 4th ed. St. Louis, MO, Mosby, pp 1–50

37. Brand PW (1983) The diabetic foot. In: Ellenberg M, Rifkin H (eds) Diabetes mellitus: theory and practice, 3rd ed. New Hyde Park, NY, Med Exam, pp 829–849
38. Müller MJ, Diamond JE, Sinacore DR, Delitto A, Blair III VP, Drury DA, Rose SJ (1989) Total contact casting in treatment of diabetic plantar ulcers. Controlled clinical trial. Diabetes Care 12:384–388
39. Edmonds ME (1987) Experience in a multidisciplinary diabetic foot clinic. In: Connor H, Boulton AJM, Ward JD (eds) The foot in diabetes. John Wiley & Sons Ltd, Chichester New York Brisbone Toronto Singapore, pp 121–133
40. Assal JP, Muklhauser I, Pernat A, Gfeller R, Jorgens V, Berger M (1985) Patient education as the basis for diabetes care in clinical practice. Diabetologia 28:602–613

## *Commentary*

*Michael Edmonds*

The chapter by Krone and Müller-Wieland has described the problems of the diabetic foot and their management. In this commentary on their chapter, four main topics will be discussed:

1. The importance of the various aetiological factors in the development of foot ulceration.
2. The place of the pressure index and arteriography in the investigation of the diabetic foot.
3. The role of antibiotic therapy in management.
4. The organisation of diabetic foot care.

### *Aetiological Factors*

Three main factors lead to tissue necrosis in the diabetic foot: neuropathy, infection and ischaemia. Infection is rarely a sole factor but complicates either neuropathy or ischaemia. Diabetic foot problems can be usually divided into those in which neuropathy predominates (neuropathic foot) and those where occlusive vascular disease is the main factor, though neuropathy may also be present in a variable degree (neuro-ischaemic foot). It is important to understand this classification, as the underlying pathology, the nature and course of the disease and its management are quite distinct in neuropathic and neuro-ischaemic feet. Neuropathy results in a warm, numb, dry and usually painless foot in which the pulses are palpable. Its characteristic feature is the plantar neuropathic ulcer. In contrast the ischaemic foot is usually cold and the pulses are absent. It is complicated by rest pain, ulceration from localized pressure necrosis and gangrene.

The presence of neuropathy is a pre-requisite for the development of the highly characteristic lesions when the circulation is intact. At the very least, the small nerve fibres are damaged causing diminished thermal and pain sensation [1] and sympathetic denervation leading to an increased peripheral circulation [2] and diminished or absent sweating. Loss of other sensory modalities is usually demonstrable as well, and the feet are sometimes anaesthetic; but occasionally a dissociated sensory loss is observed with intact large fibre modalities (vibration perception and light touch) [3]. Sympathetic denervation leads to abnormal vascular responses in the neuropathic foot [4]. Apart from a limitation of maximal blood flow in response to heating, there is a marked diminution of vasoconstriction in the dependent foot or following a sympathetic stimulus [5]. The presence of substantial arteriovenous shunting might in theory jeopardise capillary nutritional blood flow. New methods of examination show that this is not the case. Measurement of capillary blood flow by laser Doppler flowmetry shows overall a higher flow than normal and this is further confirmed by direct visualisation of capillary blood flow velocity using television microscopy [6].

Neuropathic ulcers result from mechanical, thermal and chemical injuries, in the presence of an intact circulation. The most common cause is neglected callosities which develop at sites of high vertical and shear forces under the plantar surface. These forces are determined by structural deformities in the neuropathic foot.

*Ischaemia*

The main factor responsible for a reduction in blood supply to the foot is atherosclerosis of the large vessels of the leg which in the diabetic is often multisegmental, bilateral and distal, involving tibial and peroneal vessels [7]. The actual histopathology of the large vessel wall is similar to that in non-diabetics. Fatty deposits occur in plaques within the intima. The plaques are most commonly localized at bifurcations, on the posterior walls of arteries and where the arteries are compressed by muscle fascia as in the adductor canal [8].

So-called small vessel disease involving capillaries and arterioles has been thought to contribute substantially to impaired circulation in the feet. However, the significance of obliterative lesions of arterioles and capillaries with endothelial proliferation and basement membrane thickening is not known and the role if any in the development of lesions remains to be elucidated [9].

Previous emphasis on small vessel disease has led to misconceptions in the diabetic foot with inappropriate care and therapeutic nihilism. Three misconceptions need comment.

1. Tissue necrosis that is secondary to infection is often blamed on microangiopathy. This is often not true and sepsis is therefore not treated with appropriate antibiotic therapy.
2. The value of arterial reconstructions are questioned because it is thought that if such procedures are performed, they will be of little benefit because of microangiopathy. However, this has not been the experience of vascular surgeons [10].
3. Microangiopathy secondary to diabetes is implicated in the pathogenesis of the neuropathic ulcer. However, such lesions in the diabetic foot behave exactly the same as neuropathic ulcers in the non-diabetic such as in hereditary sensory neuropathy or traumatic nerve injuries when obviously microangiopathy is absent.

When the epithelium is damaged in the skin of the diabetic foot, infection can supervene caused by organisms from the surrounding skin which are usually *Staphylococcus aureus* or *Streptococci*. Occasionally both *Staphylococci* and *Streptococci* are present together and these can combine to produce a rampant cellulitis that extends rapidly through the foot producing marked necrosis within only a few hours. Enzymes from these bacteria are angiotoxic and cause in situ thrombosis of vessels. If both vessels are thrombosed in the toe, then it becomes necrotic and gangrenous and this is probably the basis of so called "diabetic" gangrene in which tissue necrosis is seen only a few centimetres away from a bounding dorsalis pedis pulse. Gram negative organisms and anaerobic bacteria flourish in deep seated infection.

*Investigations of the Diabetic Foot*

Measurement of systolic pressure at the ankle and derivation of the pressure index is still a very useful bedside investigation in the diabetic, despite 5–10% of diabetics having stiff non-compressible peripheral vessels. The pressure index is valuable in confirming a clinical classification of the foot into neuropathic or neuroischaemic. In the former the pulses are palpable and the pressure index greater than 1.0, whereas in the neuro-ischaemic foot the pulses are absent and the pressure index usually less than 1.0, unless the vessels are calcified. This will be obvious from an artefactually high ankle pressure of greater than 200 mm Hg.

Arteriography is the investigation of choice in the neuroischaemic foot and is indicated when there is intractable rest pain and ulceration that does not respond to medical treatment. Arteriography should rarely be needed in the neuropathic foot. If a neuropathic ulcer proves indolent, then it is usually because of underlying osteomyelitis. In a series of 148 patients with neuropathic ulcers, 204/238 ulcers were healed by conservative measures. The remainder needed local surgery to drain pus or remove a "ray". All patients had palpable pulses and none needed arteriography [11].

*Management of the Diabetic Foot: Role of Antibiotics*

A bacterial swab should be taken from the floor of the ulcer after debridement. In the Diabetic Foot Clinic at King's College Hospital antibiotics are given routinely to all foot ulcers until they are healed, not only to treat existing infection if present but also to prevent further secondary infection. If a particular organism is isolated from the swab, appropriate antibiotics are given. If the swab is negative then penicillin V and flucloxacillin are prescribed to prevent infection by *Staphylococcus aureus* and *Streptococci*. If definite cellulitis or abscess is present, then urgent hospital admission is arranged and appropriate intravenous antibiotics are given according to the results of bacterial cultures.

*Organisation of Diabetic Foot Care – The Diabetic Foot Clinic*

It is vital that there is close liaison between chiropodist, shoe fitter, physician and surgeon in the care of the diabetic foot and since 1981 diabetic foot problems have been treated within a special Diabetic Foot Clinic at King's College Hospital [11]. It has provided intensive chiropody, close surveillance and prompt treatment of foot infection, and a footwear service by the attending shoe-fitter. Essential aspects of management are the provision of specially constructed shoes, intensive chiropody and precise antibiotic therapy.

The effect of the foot clinic on the number of major amputations and minor operations (which comprised drainage operations and "ray" amputations) was assessed by comparing the number of such procedures in both neuropathic and ischaemic patients from the diabetic clinic for two years prior to the establishment of the foot clinic to those performed for three years after. In the two years prior to the clinic, there were 11 and 12 major amputations each year. This was reduced in the three years following its establishment to seven, seven and five amputations respectively. Similarly the number of minor operations was also reduced from 27 and 29 yearly before the clinic to 16, 21 and 15 per year after its establishment.

## *References*

1. Guy RJG, Clark CA, Malcolm PN, Watkins PJ (1985) Evaluation of thermal and vibration sensation in diabetic neuropathy. Diabetologia 28:131
2. Edmonds ME, Roberts VC, Watkins PJ (1982) Blood flow in the diabetic neuropathic foot. Diabetologia 27:563
3. Jamal GA, Weir AI, Hansen S, Ballantyne JP (1985) An improved automated method for the measurement of thermal thresholds in patients with peripheral neuropathy. J Neurol Neurosurg Psychiat 48:361
4. Tooke JE (1987) The microcirculation in diabetes. Diabetic Medicine 4:189
5. Flynn MD (Personal communication)
6. Flynn MD, Tooke JE, Watkins PJ (1986) Abnormal capillary blood flow in the diabetic neuropathic foot, assessed by direct television microscopy. Diabetic Medicine 3:587A
7. Strandness DE Jr, Priest RE, Gibbons GE (1964) Combined clinical and pathologic study of diabetic and non diabetic peripheral arterial disease. Diabetes 13:166
8. Wheelock FC, Gibbons GW, Marble A (1985) Surgery in diabetes. In: Marble A, Krall LP, Bradley RF, Christlieb AR, Soeldner HS (eds) Joslin's diabetes mellitus. Lea and Febiger, Philadelphia, p 712
9. Logerfo FW, Coffman JD (1984) Vascular and microvascular disease of the foot in diabetes. New England Journal of Medicine 311:1615
10. Jacobs RL, Karmody A (1982) The diabetic foot. In: Jahss MH (ed) Disorders of the foot. WB Saunders Company, Philadelphia, p 1377
11. Edmonds ME, Blundell MP, Morris HE et al. (1986) Improved survival of the diabetic foot: the role of a special foot clinic. Quarterly Journal of Medicine 232:736

# Chapter 11

## Conclusions

John Dormandy and Günter Stock

"Man is as old as his arteries" and the arteries of men with critical leg ischaemia are very old. The foot with pain all night or the ulcerated leg is only a local manifestation of a generalised disease which, by similar processes in the heart or brain, will lead to irreversible ischaemia and death. Treating such patients with severe leg ischaemia is unglamorous and ultimately a losing battle, which is partly the reason it has been a relatively neglected field in medicine. We are unaware of another book directed solely at the care of these patients from a multidisciplinary point of view. Yet such patients are common, although the absence of precise figures matches our previous neglect. A best guess puts the incidence at approximately 1000/million population/year. Although their life expectancy may be short, it is surely worth while to try and maintain the quality of their remaining life. The treatment of critical limb ischaemia is aimed at trying to help these patients to continue their life with two painless legs.

The Consensus process on which this book is based began in 1988, bringing together the expertise from the many disciplines which have been treating the various aspects of critical leg ischaemia. The process began with a series of specialist workshops. Their outcome was then discussed in March 1989 by 120 specialists in the basic sciences, angiology, cardiology, diabetes, interventional radiology and vascular surgery (Fig. 1). The result was the first Consensus Document on the Pathophysiology and Management of Critical Limb Ischaemia (Fig. 1).

Expert consensus meetings and consensus views have mushroomed in the last few years; and very welcome they are. The consensus on critical ischaemia is perhaps different from most in that it aims to be a dynamic and continuously evolving process with a long term commitment by increasing numbers of expert participants. Given the large lacunae in our knowledge about this condition, the consensus view has to keep pace with increasing new pathological and clinical information. During 1990 the first Consensus Document will be reviewed and updated by seven European specialist groups. Representatives of these societies will then come together in 1991, two years after the original Consensus Meeting, and arrive at what will hopefully be an expanded, updated and revised Consensus Document II (Fig. 2).

Inevitably the consensus view was impersonal and could not include detailed exposition, argument and references. To overcome these drawbacks, this book

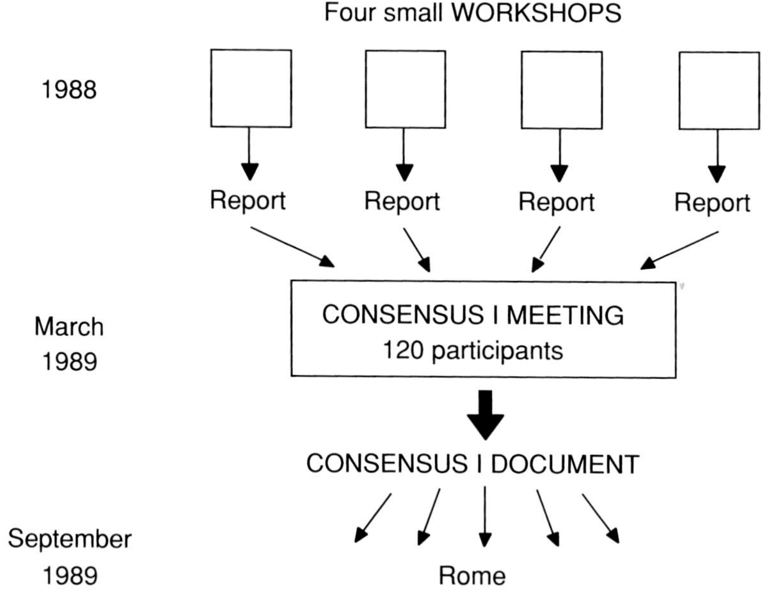


**Fig. 1.** The Consensus process – so far

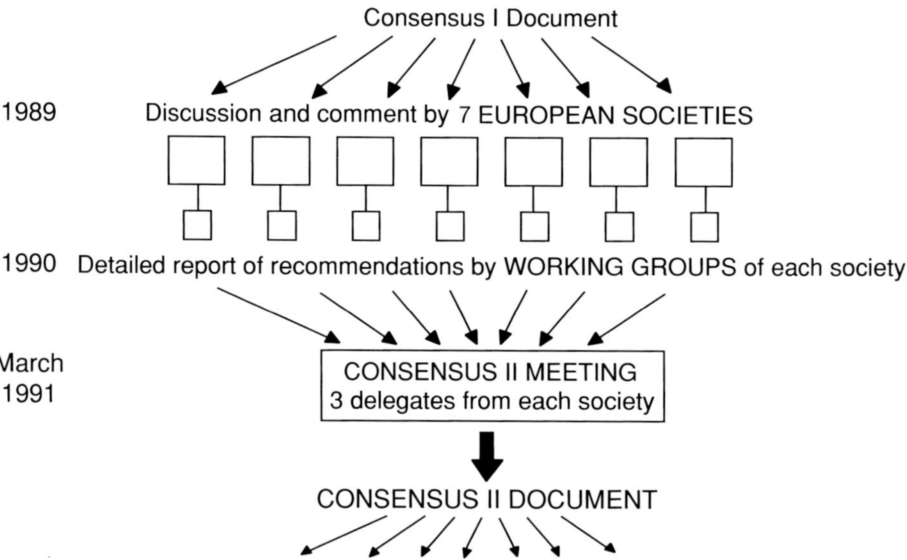


**Fig. 2.** The Consensus process – the next phase

has been written as a companion volume, where the consensus recommendations are juxtaposed with the personal views of the authors of the individual chapters, the majority of whom were also participants at the Consensus Meeting. To give some of the flavour of the discussions which took place at that meeting, one or more commentators were asked to contribute their own views at the end of each chapter.

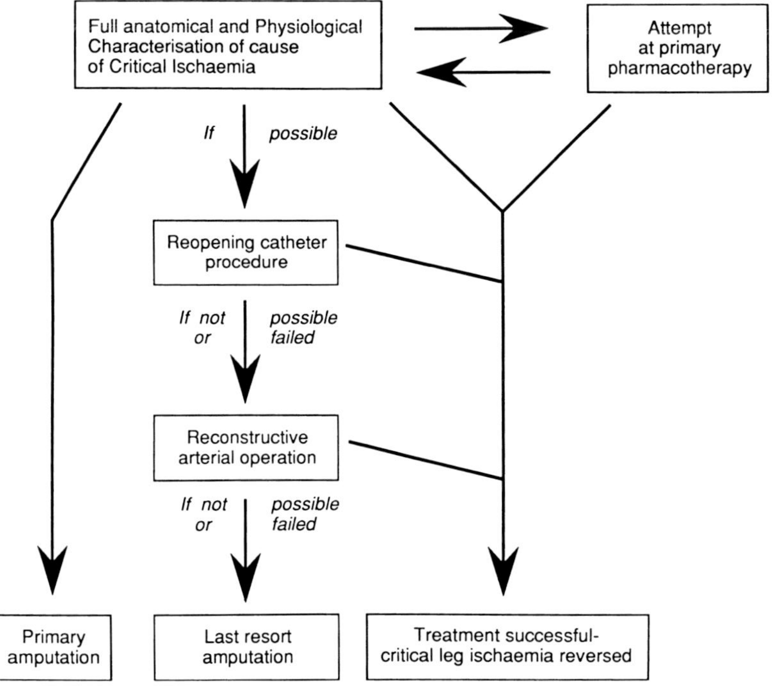


**Fig. 3.** An overall management policy of patients with critical leg ischaemia

Progress in the management of critical leg ischaemia must be based on an improved understanding of its pathophysiology, as much of our present treatment is still very empirical. Surgeons bypass occluded arteries, but on a fundamental level know little why so many bypasses fail, let alone why sometimes an anatomically successful bypass fails to reverse the distal microscopic process. Similarly, interventional radiologists dilate occlusions and stenoses, but know little of the mechanism of rethrombosis. The essential microcirculatory changes that need to be the target for successful pharmacotherapy are equally shrouded in conjecture. The concepts of microvascular flow regulating (MFR) and microvascular defence systems (MDS), with deregulation of the former and inappropriate activation of the latter are useful hypotheses, as it systematises a large number of described phenomena. It is however still largely based on indirect clinical and experimental animal findings. What happens at the cellular or microcirculatory level in critically ischaemic tissues can only be guessed on the basis of fragmented information from capillaroscopy, transcutaneous oxygen tension measurements and a range of haematological and biochemical tests usually on venous blood drawn at a distance from the ischaemic region.

An overall management policy of patients with critical leg ischaemia is illustrated in Fig. 3. It emphasises the four primary options which may be taken, having optimised the general cardio-respiratory status of the patients. In addition to the obvious and well-trodden pathway of trying to correct the major arterial occlusion by a catheter or surgical procedure, there are three other alternatives which should be considered at an early stage: The possibility that by improving the patient's cardiac output and oxygenation, the critical ischaemia may be controlled, at least for a time. Primary amputation, for cases where a major amputation is probably inevitable and is best performed as quickly as possible. Finally, the possibility of improving the ischaemic distal microcirculation by some form of effective targetted primary pharmacotherapy. One of the most urgent problems in the management of these patients is the absence of reliable proven guidelines for making these choices. It is this area which will be addressed in particular during the development of the next Consensus Document (Consensus Document II).

Multidisciplinary approach is a popular catchword, often remaining merely an empty proclamation of good intent. Being an expert is often synonymous with being an individualist, who does not take kindly to true collaborative efforts. Perhaps the most serious casualty of the widespread surgical bias in the management of critical ischaemia is the failure to optimise the general cardiorespiratory status of the patients. Vascular surgeons, like every other specialist, want to do what they are best at; that is reconstructing arteries. Yet it is the frequent experience of many cardiologists and angiologists that improving the cardiac output and respiratory function and reducing the local oedema tips many patients with critical ischaemia back into a painless and, at least temporarily, functional state. Similarly, too often patients are treated medically without referral to a surgeon until the patient is too ill and the distal circulation too compromised for any form of arterial reconstruction.

Whilst collaboration between the surgeon and internist is often made difficult in practice by the traditional separation of hospital departments, liaison between either and the interventional radiologist is easier because of the historical role of radiology as a service department. But perhaps even this is going to break down with the increasing habit of direct referral of patients to interventional radiologists. This is perhaps understandable, as undoubtedly the greatest advance in the "re-plumbing" of blocked arteries during the past decade has come from catheter reopening procedures by radiologists, rather than any new operative techniques or graft materials. Unfortunately the amazing ingenuity of new reboring techniques has not been matched by the necessary corollary of maintaining patency in the reopened arteries. There have been surprisingly few prospective controlled studies of adjuvant pharmacotherapy following peripheral angioplasty. Devising yet more ingenious techniques for percutaneous reopening procedures will have to be matched by improved post-reopening pharmacotherapy.

This central problem is not dissimilar in reconstructive vascular surgery, where surgeons can technically construct bypasses to ever more distal and narrower arteries, but early as well as late graft thrombosis is often so high that it is difficult to justify the attempt. While there is agreement that some form of postoperative pharmacotherapy is necessary in distal grafts, there are few if any good studies to show which of the currently available types of drug is best. One of the most puzzling anomalies highlighted by the interdisciplinary approach of the consensus process is the contrast in the level of evidence necessary for using a new drug and a new operation. The rigorous prospective randomised controlled study which any new drug is expected to undergo, quite rightly, is yet to be required of a new, let alone an "established", operation. More often than not, arguments for a new procedure are based on comparison with historical controls, often not even in the same centre. Large, properly designed and monitored studies would seem to be particularly appropriate as an operation is much less reproducible than the pharmacological action of a drug; each surgical "pill" is different from the next even if administered by the same surgeon. The fact that such proper surgical trials are difficult to organise and would take a long time has probably stopped doctors as well as the regulatory authorities from requiring then on behalf of new surgical approaches. There are of course special problems in any large multi-centre trial of a surgical procedure; for instance an operation, even within a single centre, will never be quite the same, nor can it be performed blind in the sense that a pill can be administered double-blind. It is in this context the first recommendation of the Consensus Document should be most taken to heart: "It is recommended that all units dealing with critical limb ischaemia should maintain accurate audited records of patients treated and their progress". The decision whether to perform a particular limb salvage operation in a particular centre should depend on the results obtained in that same centre. Too often, operations are justified on the basis of results published by an enthusiastic group who devised the technique, often in another country.

No surgeon likes to perform an amputation. An amputation is not usually seen as a success; at best it can avoid being yet another failure by healing well. Unfortunately, approximately one in three below-knee amputations do not heal primarily and half of these have to be re-amputated above the knee. Again, there have been no proper trials of adjuvant pharmacotherapy aimed at improving the healing of more distal amputations. In an attempt to avoid amputation, too many patients with critical leg ischaemia linger in hospital for months, with fruitless attempts at limb salvage reconstruction, trials of ineffective pharmacotherapy and unrealistically distal amputations, before they finally leave the hospital too bed-bound ever to rehabilitate. The opposite attitude, possibly leading to unnecessarily high amputations, may prevail in some non-specialised centres. Bernard Shaw, revealing his usual profound scepticism for the motive of doctors, said,

"It cannot be too often repeated than when an operation is once performed, nobody can ever prove that it was unnecessary. If I refuse to allow my leg to be amputated, its mortification and my death may prove that I was wrong; but if I let the leg go, nobody can ever prove that it would not have mortified had I been obstinate. Operation is therefore the safe side for the surgeon ..."

Unfortunately, there are no guidelines or tests which will accurately predict which patient should have an early primary amputation with rapid rehabilitation, rather than attempts at limb salvage. In the area of assessment and diagnosis, this is probably the most urgent question that needs to be answered. Hopefully, the developing Consensus process will in due course arrive at such guidelines.

The preferred ideal solution to the problem of treating critical leg ischaemia would be some form of pharmacotherapy which could hold in check the local ischaemia, allowing the patient to finish his life on two painless legs. The published evidence does not yet suggest that such a drug is available on the market, although some of the early results with prostanoids show promise. For the moment primary pharmacotherapy for critical limb ischaemia is only being tested in patients who have already failed or are completely unsuitable for any surgical or percutaneous catheter procedures. This is perhaps unfair and illogical. If a drug may truly prevent a significant number of major amputations it should be tested in a randomised study against surgery and angioplasty in all patients with critical limb ischaemia.

After participating in the Consensus process so far and reading the reports and commentaries of the two dozen experts in this book, there are two overwhelming conclusions to be drawn. Firstly, although many patients' critical limb ischaemia is successfully treated by currently available techniques of arterial surgery and percutaneous catheter procedures, a substantial proportion still require major amputations, even in the best specialised centres. Secondly, compared with other manifestations of circulatory disease, for instance hypertension, claudication or angina, far less basic and clinical research has been applied to the field of critical limb ischaemia. The most neglected area is pharmacotherapy, both primary and adjuvant; a reflection no doubt of the existing pre-eminent surgical bias in the management of critical ischaemia. It is the principal purpose of the ongoing Consensus process to try and remedy these problems.

# Subject Index